Chronicling a Crisis

Chronicling a Crisis

SUNY Oneonta's Pandemic Diaries

Edited by

ED BECK, DARREN D. CHASE,
MATTHEW C. HENDLEY, and ANN A. TRAITOR

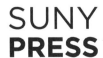

SUNY
PRESS

Cover image: © Jessica Rothman

Published by State University of New York Press, Albany

Printed in the United States of America

For information, contact State University of New York Press, Albany, NY
www.sunypress.edu

Library of Congress Cataloging-in-Publication Data

Names: Beck, Ed, 1987– editor. | Chase, Darren, 1969– editor. | Hendley,
    Matthew, 1966– editor. | Traito, Ann A., 1966– editor.
Title: Chronicling a crisis : SUNY Oneonta's pandemic diaries / edited by
    Ed Beck, Darren Chase, Matthew C. Hendley, and Ann A. Traito.
Other titles: State University of New York Oneonta's pandemic diaries
Description: Albany : State University of New York Press, [2023] | Includes
    bibliographical references and index.
Identifiers: LCCN 2023009085 | ISBN 9781438495316 (hardcover : alk. paper) |
    ISBN 9781438495323 (ebook) | ISBN 9781438495309 (pbk. : alk. paper)
Subjects: LCSH: State University of New York College at Oneonta—History. |
    College students—New York (State)—Social conditions. | Community and
    college—New York (State)—Social conditions. | COVID-19 Pandemic,
    2020—-Influence.
Classification: LCC LB1921.O252 C47 2023 | DDC 378.747—dc23/eng/20230621
LC record available at https://lccn.loc.gov/2023009085

10 9 8 7 6 5 4 3 2 1

Contents

Part IV. Winter 2020–21

Part V. Spring 2021

Prologue

MATTHEW C. HENDLEY AND ANN A. TRAITOR

What This Book Is

This book is a primary source collection of the moment, which documents and reflects on the experience of students, faculty, and staff at the State University of New York at Oneonta (SUNY Oneonta) during a global pandemic. Originally founded in 1889, SUNY Oneonta is a comprehensive four-year public college of about 6,500 students in the State University of New York system located in Oneonta, New York. This book, *Chronicling a Crisis: SUNY Oneonta's Pandemic Diaries* (based on an online collaborative blog, *The Semester of Living Dangerously*) was inspired by Mass Observation, a maverick experiment launched in Britain during the 1930s to gather written public observations of everyday life. Mass Observation has become an invaluable set of primary sources for researchers trying to delve into the social history of Britain between 1937 and 1950. Our project grew from a class assignment to a blog to the book you hold in your hands. Its story begins below.

Origin Story

How did the inspiration from a century-old UK popular history project lead to this book? Some years ago, Ann Traitor, a longtime adjunct professor at SUNY Oneonta, was in an airport in Denmark. Already tired from a long overnight flight and with a seven-hour layover ahead of her, she hit the airport bookstore. After locating the English language section, she found a book called *Our Longest Days*, a selection of wartime diary entries taken from the archives of the Mass Observation, a project founded in the UK in 1937. Ann had heard of Mass Observation but had never worked with or read its material before. In her tired state, the book seemed to hit all the marks: it was historical, it was reasonably priced, and it was a selection of diary entries—easy for the tired brain to make sense of, and the dated entries made clear stopping points.

Ann's traveling companions were nonplussed (she had also gotten a stack of newspapers that seemed more fun, which they quickly commandeered), so she began to read the book, more to stay awake than out of any real enthusiasm. There were still five and a half hours of "layover" to go, after all. She began the book hoping to pass the time, but then found she couldn't put it down. She devoured the book and had finished it by the time the plane landed at its final destination. She immediately made plans to incorporate sections of it in one of her courses at SUNY Oneonta.

The first class discussion she had about Mass Observation was in her Western Civilization II class. It was so lively that Ann had to ask the students to tone down the shouting. The students were quite animated in their response to one diarist in particular, the teenaged Muriel Green. A girl who worked in the Women's Land Army, Muriel's entries reflected the difficulty of simultaneously being a nineteen-year-old on the lookout for fun and being a serious war worker on the home front, responsible for growing the food that would feed the nation. When asked if Muriel's entries represented "life though a war lens" or "war though a life lens," the classroom erupted. Some students vehemently replied that they saw Muriel as too frivolous, too worried about dancing with soldiers, and too worried about her looks! Others just as vehemently replied that they saw Muriel as seriously shouldering the responsibility of being a "Land Girl" as she religiously got up early to plant, weed, or harvest, day in and day out, no matter the weather. Muriel deserved to write about a little bit of fun or she would have gone crazy! That was when the shouting began.

Fast-forward, if you will, to the spring of 2020, the COVID Spring. All the college students were sent home and the faculty members were now furiously working to move all of their course content online and figure out how to teach the remaining material virtually. There was not much time, a week at most, and the rules kept changing and the various problems kept coming, everything from weak internet signals to students with no computers.

In the flurry of moving all of Ann's lectures and assignments to an online, non–face-to-face format, she realized that one of her assignments, the fun map quiz of Europe, was just too "low tech" to be online. It consisted of a photocopied blank map of Europe with ten countries randomly chosen for identification. How in the world could that be done online? While she was madly searching the internet, looking for some kind of customizable map quiz that was not geared for elementary students—"color France pink!"—she lamented the absence of another assignment that would lend itself to an online format. It is safe to say Ann was at her maximum point of frustration.

At that moment, two things happened: one of Ann's favorite quotes from Anton Chekhov popped into her head: "Any idiot can survive a crisis; it's this day-to-day living that wears you out." "True," Ann thought, "but what happens when your daily life *is* the crisis? Then what?" In the very next instant, she thought, "If it is this tough for me, and I have some experience of online teaching, what in the world must be going through the students' minds?How must they be feeling right now?" That is when she thought of the diary project. Like a bolt out of the blue, Mass Observation came to mind. Why not create her own version of Mass Observation? This seemed a perfect time: our day-to-day living was certainly a crisis, and this project might help students manage the crisis, to get them to think about what they are experiencing right now, to allow them to view themselves as part of a larger moment, to relieve some stress by letting paper take some of the weight, . . . and also to get a little extra credit for the class. Ann then approached the chair of SUNY Oneonta's History Department, Dr. Matthew C. Hendley, wondering if this idea could be opened up to all history majors, giving them a chance to help create those "first-person," eyewitness narratives that always make for compelling reading? As a postdoctoral fellow, Matthew had done primary research in the Mass Observation archive at the University of Sussex in the 1990s, and was thinking along similar lines. He had already been actively pondering how SUNY Oneonta's students and faculty might document this unprecedented crisis. Consequently, Matthew most enthusi-astically embraced Ann's creative idea and applauded her vision. Ann and Matthew decided that they would take physical items of any kind—paper diaries, artwork, pictures—as well as anything electronically sent. Originally the project was to be restricted to history students only, but then it grew.

Matthew approached the director of SUNY Oneonta's college library, Darren D. Chase, to see about making an archive at the college for any paper-based materials that might be submitted. The project mushroomed from there. The next idea was to open it up to more than just history students, as the entire campus was also living though this moment in crisis, in their own various ways. In order to maximize participation, Darren and Matthew thought it could be expanded into a blog. Darren then brought Ed Beck, an instructional designer from SUNY Oneonta's Teaching, Technology and Learning Center, into the picture. Ed is responsible for the attractive blog format using WordPress, its user-friendliness, and a host of other inventive ideas. It is from this sequence of unforeseen events and convergences that the blog and later this book were born.

Why SUNY Oneonta?

Scenically located on the rolling foothills of the Catskill Mountains between Albany and Binghamton, SUNY Oneonta appeared to be an idyllic location in which to study and live. Thoughts of worldwide pandemics never ordinarily entered the thoughts of this college community. COVID changed everything. As this book will show, SUNY Oneonta had a unique experience that is worthy of documentation and consideration. New York State was the original epicenter of the COVID pandemic in the US. The pandemic hit New York City early and hard, and it then rapidly spread throughout the rest of the state and eventually the entire country. SUNY Oneonta was naturally affected by the statewide catastrophe. About 40 percent of its student body hails from "Downstate" New York (i.e., New York City, Long Island, and Hudson Valley), and the remainder are from Upstate New York. The nature of our student body meant that these statewide health developments impacted the campus directly. Further, SUNY Oneonta itself had several crucial milestones. It was the only college in New York State that had to send its students home twice (spring 2020 semester and fall 2020). The fall 2020 outbreak was especially severe, leading to almost 500 students testing positive within the first two weeks of class. This was the most rapid outbreak of COVID in any college in the Northeast, and received national and international media coverage. The *New York Times* included coverage in multiple articles, with pictures of college staff in Hazmat suits in the middle of the night taking pajama-clad students (who had tested positive) out of their dorms and into isolation.[1] Newspapers in the UK (including

---

1. "SUNY Oneonta Ends In-Person Classes for Fall as Outbreak Nears 400 Cases," *New York Times*, September 4, 2020, section A, p. 6.

the *Daily Mail*) and even China picked up the story.[2] SUNY Oneonta was the canary in the coal mine for college spread of COVID in the US. For a moment, all eyes were on this particular campus. All teaching had to rapidly evolve to online, hundreds of students tested positive, and thousands of lives were upended. The fear and dislocation were palpable. Eventually, SUNY Oneonta's president resigned, and a new acting president was put in place.[3] The campus stabilized and students, staff, and faculty struggled to adjust, and through mutual hard work the academic year was completed. All of this is recorded in this book.

Why Spring 2020–Spring 2021?

The COVID pandemic is a long-lasting phenomenon. When it began, few would have guessed that more than two years later at least 100,000 Americans per day would still be testing positive in June 2022. It may be years into the future before COVID finally ceases to be a public health concern. That said, the period covered in this book (spring 2020–spring 2021) is unique and noteworthy. From an academic perspective, organizing the book centrally around semesters fits the ebb and flow of campus life. From the historical perspective this also makes sense. The main crisis and most "historic" episode of the COVID crisis for SUNY Oneonta, New York State, and arguably the US, occurred between the spring 2020 and spring 2021 period. Spring 2020 was the apex of the catastrophe in which there was no vaccine, and there was mass fear, mass isolation, and mass disruption. There

---

2. Emily Crane, "Selfies, Suspensions and COVID-19 SWAT Teams: Inside the Worst College Outbreak in New York Where More than 670 students—10 percent of the campus—have tested positive," *Daily Mail*, September 18, 2020; "Ministry of Education Emergency Report: University Outbreak: 500 Students Confirmed Positive. Six Thousand Students Were Forced to Close their Classes!" *Language Journal* (September 6, 2020) (China), https://mp.weixin.qq.com/s/wjjyoNJYeVgXQzkZKMG_nA; "Can't Hold up Further? Or Is There a Hidden Story? 712 Students at a University in the United States Infected by COVID-19! Principal Resigns," Baidu.com, https://mbd.baidu.com/newspage/data/landingshare?context=%7B%22nid%22%3A%22news_9628084988275431961%22%7D&isBdboxFrom=1&pageType=1&rs=3759692922&ruk=M_IxdYGojxdGRICBgb2MXg&urlext=%7B%22cuid%22%3A%22li2p8litva_RiSuQ0ivsa_aMv80h8Hutji2d8_Pjvf0gu SaTliHRaY8XSu0Q8QPjJtEmA%22%7D.

3. Amanda Rosa, "After 700 Students Test Positive, a College President Resigns," *New York Times*, October 15, 2020.

was a sense of managed optimism in summer 2020, and the college tried to reopen in the fall. As was previously mentioned, fall 2020 started badly at SUNY Oneonta and elsewhere in the country. Nevertheless, by the end of the fall 2020 semester, vaccines were being approved. In spring 2021, vaccines began to be rolled out, and the college brought a limited number of students back with 20 percent of the classes being held in a hybrid online/in-person format and 80 percent online. By fall 2021, though COVID had not been vanquished the main crisis was over. Almost all classes were held in person and students all had to be vaccinated. Students did get ill and some went into isolation or quarantine, but "normality" or a version of it had been restored. As time moves on, it is hard to get back into the mental space of the spring 2020–spring 2021 period. For that reason, it is crucial that the hopes, fears, panic, and resilience of that time be recorded and historically preserved. As follows, we will show how a joint project emerged first as a blog and later as this book to record in words and pictures the experience of an entire college community during this time.

The Format and Organization of This Book

The organization of the book is as follows: it begins with an Introduction, followed by a curated selection of blog entries, and concludes with scholarly and supporting materials about the project. There are over 200 entries submitted between March 2020 and June 2021 by SUNY Oneonta faculty, staff, and students included in this book. Most of the entries are text-based. Some entries have text and photos. Some are images only. All entries are published with permission of their creators and are reproduced as they appeared in the blog. The entries are arranged by semester with sections for spring 2020, summer 2020, fall 2020, winter 2020–21, and spring 2021. There is a time line of key events at the campus, local, state, and national level for each month detailed in the entries. The final section includes a detailed historical analysis of the inspiration for the blog and this book—the Mass Observation Project in the UK. That section examines the evolution of Mass Observation from 1937 to the present, as well as the scholarship that has emerged from it. It concludes by analyzing key differences and similarities between the paper-based Mass Observation project and the brave new digital world represented by the SUNY Oneonta pandemic diaries. "From Pixels to Paper: Building Blog and Book" explains in greater depth the evolution of the project, the technology and concepts used to set up and run the blog, and the lessons learned from the project. "Themes" is an overview of some of the main themes that appeared in the pandemic diary entries that are reproduced in the book. Using Voyant Tools and other methods, oft-repeated themes and associated quotes from entries are highlighted.

Reading This Book

Our hope, dear reader, is that you find some gems here for yourself, lessons to use, points to ponder, compassion to absorb. Previous books that have been based on the original UK Mass Observation Project can be read in any number of ways. While it is certainly possible to read them in a linear fashion from start to finish, most readers dip in and out of the text. There is a certain fascination in zeroing in on specific regular contributors to see how they evolve and adapt to change. It can be equally rewarding to target a range of dates rather than any particular individual to see differing reflections on a particular decisive event. It can also be just as gratifying to read along at random with no specific agenda or design just for the pleasure of discovery. In such ways treasures are found and the ordinary becomes extraordinary (and vice versa!). Our task in organizing the original blog and in compiling this book was to create a primary source collection of the moment. We leave it up to the reader how best to utilize it.

Perhaps you will see portions of your COVID times reflected in the words of these writers. Perhaps you will see different worlds and times from the COVID you lived through. Perhaps you will interpret the words of these readers from this particular time and place in your own specific way. Perhaps, more excitingly, you will be moved to start a "Mass Observation"–style project of your own. The possibilities are endless. We aim to inform our readers and help record individual responses from one location during a globally significant event. We prescribe nothing specific.

What have we learned from this moment and this project? We have learned that talking to yourself is not at all a bad thing but keeping yourself company by writing is even better. It is a gift to your future self from your present one. If we offer any advice at all it is the following: Keep observing and keep writing!

Preface

One of the more original techniques used by Mass Observation was the "directive." As Dorothy Sheridan puts it, "The Directive was never a questionnaire; rather it directed the attention of the Mass-Observers to the subject area which Mass Observation was studying at any one time."[4] Below is Ann Traitor's original "directive" for our campus community. It was from this invitation that the Pandemic Diary project began and evolved into the blog, which is the basis of this book. The original title of the blog, *The Semester of Living Dangerously*, is contained in the invitation below.

The Semester of Living Dangerously

A Pandemic Diary Project for Housebound Students, Faculty, and Staff of SUNY Oneonta

Psst! Hey, you! You there, looking at your phone and computer for continuous news updates. Aren't you getting tired of reading how we are living through a major historical moment? Wouldn't you like to *make* a little history? Of course, you would! Put that phone or computer down for a few minutes and let me tell you a little story. Then I will invite you to join the History Department to make history.

We are going through a pretty uncertain time right now, but this is not the first time folks have been afraid of the unknown. I'll bet you could come up with a few times yourself, but I am thinking of the 1930s, in

---

4. Dorothy Sheridan, Brian Street, and David Bloome, *Writing Ourselves: Mass-Observation and Literary Practices* (Cresskill, NJ: Hampton Press Inc., 2000), 75.

particular. (You look smart—I am sure you are already thinking of some scary things like the Great Depression, Mussolini, the debuts of the Philly cheesesteak sandwich and the Twinkie, to name but a few.) In Great Britain, the decade of the 1930s was a turbulent one indeed, what with the abdication crisis, the Great Depression, and the war clouds gathering over Europe, so there was certainly much to write about. At the time, the British press used quite a lot of column inches to tell the British public how they (the public) felt about these and other various events. In 1936, a young anthropologist named Tom Harrisson was angered by this arrogance on the part of the papers. Working on the idea that the British press had really no idea what the average person believed, Harrisson decided to find out those beliefs for himself. He asked the people of Britain to keep diaries of what they were doing, the thoughts they had, and any reflections on any current situation, either local or international, and then send the diaries to him. Thus, was born an organization Harrisson called "Mass Observation." Eventually, there were paid observers as well as volunteer observers, all of whom wrote their diaries and sent them to the Mass Observation headquarters in London.

By 1939, the organization was well established enough to get a personal view of the war—warts and all. Topics like blackouts, army routines, death, job searches, wartime relationships, and the rationing system are just a few of the subjects to be found within its pages. It looks like exactly the sort of thing a smart-looking person like you would pick up and read. And an exciting read it is! Who doesn't like reading a good first-person account? But even *more exciting* than reading a diary is writing a diary! This is where you come in, where you get invited to make history.

Keep a Diary

Keep a diary of your coronavirus time. Diaries can be created and shared using various modalities: a physical, paper diary; entries on *The Semester of Living Dangerously Pandemic Diaries* website; or a digital document diary. In your day-to-day existence, what would you want future readers to know? What annoys you? makes you happy? frustrates you? surprises you? bores you? You can write about anything you like, about any subject you like, for as long as you like. This exercise is also a great stress buster. Don't carry your annoyances with you—let paper take the weight! One woman participating in Mass Observation wrote a lot about rationing, food in general, and trying to keep house. You can write as much or as little as you like.

Even a sentence or two is better than no sentences at all. One man wrote consistently about the barometric pressure and the weather—and that's all. One eighteen-year-old girl wrote pages and pages about boys, dances, and future prospects, all while barely mentioning the war. Give yourself the gift of reflection—take whatever time you can when you can to write whatever you can. This is your exciting opportunity to become the first-person narrative we all enjoy reading!

Whatever format you choose, we need entries—so get writing. Put aside your work and daily angst for a few minutes and write for yourself. Document this important time. You never know where a project like this might lead you! Get writing! You could create a future building block of history, or less grandiosely, have a record to show others of how you survived this truly unusual time.

The Details

You can write a physical paper diary or create an account on *The Semester of Living Dangerously* website for electronic entries. All diaries and accounts should include your name (or a pseudonym if you chose to remain anonymous), as well as your status (student, faculty, staff, administrator). Electronic accounts require an email.

All physical diaries will become part of the College's history and are archived in the Milne Library Special Collections. They will also be digitized and—along with the electronic diaries—made available on "The Semester of Living Dangerously" website.

Get Started

1. **Paper Diary**—Create a paper diary in a notebook or journal and mail it to us upon completion. Indicate if you would like your original returned, and after the library has completed digitizing it a pick-up will be scheduled.

2. **Electronic Diary**—Share your thoughts and impressions online! Simply click the "Contribute" button on *The Semester of Living Dangerously* website, and log in with your SUNY Oneonta account.

3. **Digital Document Diary**—Feel free to write your diary on a Word document or using another word-processor program.

Stop checking the news every five minutes—that time is better spent! Start writing!

Acknowledgments

We would like to thank the blog contributors, without whom *Chronicling a Crisis: SUNY Oneonta's Pandemic Diaries* would never have happened, as well as SUNY Press for making this book possible. We would like to laud Jessica Rothman's original and innovative design for our book cover, which managed to encompass the essence of our project. We would like to acknowledge one another's mutual patience and diligence throughout this entire project. Collegiality and good humor meant deadlines were met and we all continued to enjoy each other's company!

Matthew would also like to thank his family (Michelle, Jonathon, and Sara), with whom he cocooned during the pandemic, and his colleagues in SUNY Oneonta's History Department. He also would like to send a special thank you to the spirits of Charles Madge, Humphrey Jennings, and Tom Harrisson, whose original creation of the Mass Observation Project in the UK during a distant crisis-riven decade gave us the inspiration to record History as it happened.

Ann would like to send a special thank you to her family: mano mylimai dukrai, mano puikiems giminaičiams ir artimesniems ir vienam geram žmogui. She would also like to dedicate this work to all those during the pandemic who fell down seven times but got up eight. Well done you!

Darren would like to thank his beloved family (Kristina, Jordan, Parker, Kalyna, and Maksym). He dedicates this work to the staff of the James M. Milne Library, in honor of their steady commitment to SUNY Oneonta throughout the pandemic and beyond.

Ed would like to thank his wife Kristen for her support, and Tim Stookesberry, an early champion of this project.

Part I

Spring 2020

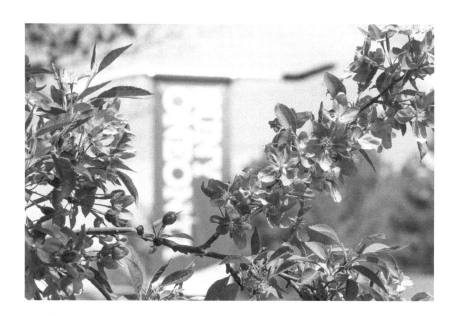

March 2020

SUNY ONEONTA

March 23—Classes transition to online formats and the campus is closed to all but a few students.

ONEONTA

March 26—Otsego County announces its first death from COVID-19.

March 30—State Senator James Seward (R Milford) and wife test positive for COVID. Senator Seward is hospitalized and placed in a medically induced coma before recovering.

NEW YORK

March 1—The first case of COVID-19 is reported in Manhattan.

March 2—New York City Mayor Bill de Blasio tells New Yorkers in a tweet to ignore the virus and continue as normal.

March 7—Governor Andrew Cuomo declares a state of emergency.

March 31—The first COVID-related death of a child is reported in New York City.

USA

March 13—President Trump declared COVID-19 a national emergency.

March 17—The death toll from COVID-19 reaches 100.

March 26—The United States officially becomes the country hardest hit by the pandemic, with at least 81,000 confirmed cases and 1,000 deaths.

WORLD

March 11—WHO declares COVID-19 a pandemic.

Diary Entries

March 24, 2020

Maggie McCann

March 24, 2020. Although this is my first entry, I am roughly a week and one day into self-quarantine with my family. I've been home from school now two and a half weeks, a week, and a half longer than anyone was expecting.

When I left for spring break on March 5th a world pandemic was nowhere on my mind, nowhere in the news, it was not a possibility. As the week went on the world seemed to change overnight. I left on Friday, by Monday schools were closing, the news was on 24/7, but it still felt temporary, a news story that would pass in a week leaving nothing but some examples of the worst and the best of humanity and a few new memes. By Friday it was practically at my doorstep. The number of cases, especially in New York, have been rising by the hundreds daily and SUNY schools are officially closed. This was not going away any time soon.

No one was prepared for this, especially my friends from school; other than me and my sister we all live no closer than an hour or two from each other. We knew we'd have to leave for summer, but we still had so much to do. Formals to go to, birthdays to celebrate and for a few of us, Julie, Karla, and so many more people I know, graduation was around the corner. My friends Julie, Katie, and Adalyne, we've all decided to faceTime once a week to keep in touch, but we're still so lonely stuck at home.

I'm away from my boyfriend too, Ryan. We had a pretty great set up living in a dorm away from each other at school, but Albany and Staten

Island are a bit farther apart. The weekend before everything really shut down, he came to visit just in case he couldn't by Monday.

He spent three days here; he tried his first New York City bagel and loved it (of course) and I got to show him my high school and he met more of my family. It was an amazing weekend, he left Monday, I have no idea when I'll get to see him again.

Monday was definitely my worst day, I couldn't look at social media, any news. I just wanted to shut out everything "COVID" "virus" "pandemic." I am incredibly overstimulated I need school to start back up because I cannot take much more of this.

March 25, 2020. Roughly day nine of self-isolation, I would have had my 8 a.m. film class today, followed by Environmental Sustainability at 9 a.m., with a break in classes after usually to go eat, shower, get ready for the day, then a 12 p.m. video production class. Usually, I'd study for the afternoon and have dinner with my friends at 7 p.m. and spend the night with Ryan until I went to sleep.

Ryan had an overnight shift last night but a few hours before he had to leave for it (the shift) the White House announced anyone who's left the NYC area within the last 14 days, this includes Ryan, must self-quarantine for two weeks. So, Ryan had to decide whether or not to go in. He's been working with the public for a few weeks now and only worked after close for the last three days, so he decided to go in. The new rule also effects whether or not I can get my things from my dorm when I'm scheduled to on Saturday.

We found out too that my friend, and my sister's boyfriend Jonathan's friend has tested positive for COVID, I had seen Jonathan the weekend Ryan came to visit, and Jonathan had seen his friend the day before so now I'm hyperaware of every time I sneeze.

I've been way busier with schoolwork than I was expecting, I'm taking a trip to Target today I think, after classes, I'm really looking forward to leaving the house. We're taking gloves and hand sanitizer with us just in case.

March 28, 2020. I picked up my things from my dorm today, the most excitement we've had in a few weeks honestly, and the farthest I've been from my house in about a month. I got to see Ryan; I'd be lying if I said there weren't any tears. I don't know when I'm going to get to see him again after today, it could be months. That's the worst part of all this, not knowing when it'll end, no countdown, it seems endless and it's only going to get worse before it gets better.

I'm happy to have my clothes back, I'd been wearing the same three outfits for the past three weeks, not that I have anything to dress up for, but a nice mix of sweatpants and leggings couldn't hurt. It's been a week since people have been moving their stuff out of their dorms, my friends across the hall have all moved their things out except for Kiara, it's a ghost town on campus, everyone's keeping their distance, getting in and out as fast as we can.

Classes have been going on for about a week now, most professors are keeping us organized and I appreciate that this was thrown on all of us at the same time, one of my classes was video production which was nearly all hands on so I haven't got anything from that class yet, not sure if I might have to drop it. Schools been keeping me busy and we're almost out of March, I've stopped watching the news, it helped a lot, nothing's getting better.

Diary Entries

March 24–30, 2020

JULIAN GOTIANGCO

March 24, 2020

Dear Diary,

In case you didn't already know, I'm home from school because of the Coronavirus. All our classes will be online now. I have a lot of mixed emotions. A lot of things that I had planned got canceled. I was going to see a Broadway show with family, but all Broadway shows got canceled. What I had been really looking forward to was a production of the musical Once Upon A Mattress in April. The cast and crew had been working hard, but unfortunately, the production got canceled. It was inevitable, but I cried, nonetheless. I did realize that I need to gain a little more perspective. This wasn't the end of the world, and I have many more opportunities left to perform. Many people are in a way worse situation than I am because of this virus. I had to be considerate of those people. Another big takeaway is that I made so many friends during musical rehearsals. They made me feel welcome when I was afraid that I wouldn't be welcomed. I miss them all so much. But the big takeaway for me is that I get to spend more time with my family. In the last few days, we've had movie nights, family game nights, and went on walks in the park (we're sure to follow social distancing practices). It feels weird. I can't greet my parents the way I used to when they come back from their shifts in the hospital. No hugs. No kisses or high-fives. Just a mere elbow bump or a wave. It's not the same.

I had a weird epiphany lately. I'm getting ahead of myself here. I'm looking forward to the end of the school year, but when the summer break ends, for the first time, I'm not going to be upset that I'll be going back to school. This is really the first time I can say I miss school and I wish I could be there. Classes started yesterday. I'll put in another entry when this first week is over.

March 30, 2020

Dear Diary,

We have entered week 2 of distance learning. Things are going fine so far. I got a great grade on a Calculus exam that I took last week. So that made me happy. Many of my friends seem to be using Zoom rather than Blackboard to communicate with teachers and each other. Today I was invited to my first Zoom conference, but it wasn't for school; it was for a club that I am a part of at school called Mask and Hammer. This club is geared towards anyone interested in theater like me. We usually hold meetings on Monday, and the club president wanted to try using Zoom to hold a meeting. So, I joined the video conference, and I was so happy to see my friends again, whom I all missed very much. We discussed plans of still holding the club's annual end-of-year party through Zoom even though we would not be in the same room. I met my friends' pets, which made me smile but also jealous because I do not have a pet of my own. I have also checked up on my friends from high school. I had a long conversation with my friend Vic and told her I missed her very much and that I hope she is safe with her family. Then I said something I have not really told anyone else. I worry a lot about my parents. My parents are both nurses, so they are the essential workers who are allowed out of the house to work. My parents always come home tired, and they tell me that it is frightening working in the hospital now because they had never seen anything like the coronavirus before. One day my dad planned to get the family breakfast, but he had to stay extra hours in the ER. I was afraid something happened to him, but he came home just happy to see me and the rest of my family, and I was happy to see that he was doing fine. Well, that's it for now.

March Diary Entries

March 25, 2020

Cassandra Snow

March 25, 2020

Today I didn't really do much, but I did get a lot of homework done and I am like 3 weeks ahead of homework. I sometimes think I won't finish all my homework in time, so I panic and do it all really early. I guess it is kind of a good thing and a bad thing! I also had my HUEC class, and it is always hard to focus because I really do not enjoy that class. I hate being inside and home with my sister. My parents even asked me to start dinner, which I did but didn't really want to do. I think we are having chicken parm for dinner, which is really exciting! I cannot believe the school gave us an extra week of spring break.

March 26, 2020

Today I woke up for my Nutrition class online and learned a lot. I really enjoy that class, but it was better in person since it is a very hands-on class. I also started one of my papers for my orchestra class which I'm not too happy about because I can't seem to get to the word limit, but I will work on it! It's not due until May so I have time! I'm super bored and I have trouble falling asleep because I don't do much during the day so I'm not really using energy. My mom suggested working out in the basement but no thanks!

March 29, 2020

Today I went back to school to get all my stuff. It didn't take very long but I didn't realize how much stuff I had in my room. I was also the last one to move out and it was so sad! I forgot to take my roommate's stuff she forgot out of her drawer, but she said it was okay. I still feel terrible though. We also made sure we used hand sanitizer after we finished cleaning my room. My RA was also moving out, so I got to say goodbye to him! We were going to get Chinese food for dinner, but no one answered so we made pasta and meatballs for dinner! It was so good.

March 30, 2020

Today I woke up at like 9 am which was so weird because I never get up that early. I took a shower and did some homework. I also made myself a healthy breakfast because I was bored. I took a break and watched some Netflix and then I went to class and put some of my clothes away since I just got all my clothes back from college. I also watched an episode of this show "Elite" with my boyfriend.

2

April 2020

SUNY ONEONTA

April 28—City of Oneonta Mayor Gary Herzig sends letter to Governor Cuomo requesting that college students all receive COVID tests when they return to campus again.

ONEONTA

April 7—State Senator James Seward (R Milford) moved out of intensive care while still recovering from COVID.

April 7—The General Clinton Canoe Regatta is canceled for 2020.

NEW YORK

April 10—All New York state residents are allowed to request absentee ballots for voting due to COVID.

April 15—State residents are ordered to wear face masks in public places where social distancing is not possible.

April 22—Governor Cuomo announces that the state would be starting a contact tracing program in coordination with New Jersey and Connecticut.

USA

April 2—It is reported that 10 million Americans are out of work and 6.6 million people applied for unemployment benefits in the last week of March.

WORLD

April 2—More than 1 million people were sickened with COVID-19 in 171 countries, with at least 51,000 deaths.

April 6—British Prime Minister Boris Johnson moved into intensive care, ten days after going public with the virus.

April 26—More than 2.8 million people sickened worldwide, with the global death toll surpassing 200,000.

Careful and Precise

April 1, 2020

DARREN D. CHASE

This is my diary.

It's a bright, chilly early spring day. It's April 1. A day to celebrate tricks and pranks. I'm outwitted and deceived and it's OK. It's fun to be fooled, sometimes. On the other side of midnight is April 2. Today moves into tomorrow.

What is on the other side of the pandemic? I'm hopeful and worried about what the answer includes.

I wash my hands for myself and for everyone around me. I wash them thoroughly for at least 20 seconds. Careful, precise actions are impactful. My hands are so dry and so clean. I think I remember my last handshake.

When we teleconference, I wonder about the rooms of my colleagues. Are their rooms warm or cool? Do they smell like fresh brewed coffee? Are my colleagues alone in their rooms, or are others with them out of frame?

Diary Entries

April 1, 2020

Maggie McCann

April 1, 2020. We've made it. We're out of March. The yearlong month. I cannot believe it's only April. Both the passing of days and the world outside have slowed to a snail's pace, or at least in the city it has. I can imagine things are feeling a bit less apocalyptic outside the city and New Jersey. We're seriously in the epicenter here and every day I hear of a new person, a friend of a friend, a coworker's aunt, a sister's boyfriend, all testing positive. It is creeping closer and closer.

I left my house for the first time in four days today. It is starting to get nice out so we're taking walks, my family and I. We took a ride down to Lemon Creek Park. It's the best my family and I have gotten along in days. My dad has started working every other day at work so we're all starting to get exceedingly stir crazy and were taking it out on each other. But today we went on a walk. The birds were all nesting in the group of birdhouses in the park and we spent a while watching those. We re-created a picture of my sister, my dad and I from maybe ten years ago, and we walked the beach for about a half hour. My parents told me about an old factory that used to sit right on the water, they hung out there with their friends in the '80s until it burned to the ground in '97.

We stopped by my grandparents' house, we stood at the curb while my grandparents barely stepped out of their doorway. The one thing everyone keeps asking is "Are you going to the store?" or "Do you need something from the store?" This time it was my grandma asking my mom for detergent, coffee, and paper towels (if there were any). We stood and talked for a while until we all went back home.

April 6, 2020. It's my cousin's birthday today, she's turning 19. We would usually have had a big party at her house, lots of food, lots of alcohol. Today we drove by at 4 p.m. and wished her a happy birthday from our car window. It was a beautiful day today too, we would've been out in her backyard until two in the morning, my Aunt barbecuing, my Uncle keeping the fire going, I probably would've invited Ryan down, I'm looking forward to bringing him to a family barbecue, this summer we'll probably be having one every weekend to make up for this.

Or maybe not. Going to the store today to pick up a card for Steph, I didn't even get out of the car, everyone was wearing masks, I wouldn't've gotten close to anyone, but the fear of being in a public place was enough to keep me put. What happens when this is all over, will we ever be comfortable to hug each other again? Hold the door for a stranger? Maybe we'll have parties again, we might go to movies like we used to, but things won't feel the same. There's no problem with being a bit more cautious, if we want to keep gloves on hand why don't we, but I don't know if we'll be able to socialize the way we all used to, not if this goes on for much longer.

I miss Ryan a lot, we've been Skyping quite a bit, almost every other day, he's still working at the supermarket, he's been busier than ever, he stocks so thankfully he's in the back, not working with customers. I haven't been in a store in about three weeks, I don't know what they look like now. I can't wait to see him again, I can't wait to see my friends from school either, we've been Skyping once a week, we've not much to talk about other than what we wish we were doing and what we have to do instead. We've all taken up hobbies, I picked up my guitar again, Julie's taking extra cello lessons. Grace has been drawing a bunch more and just ordered strings for her Ukulele, and if all those hobbies fail to keep us entertained, I've been trying to lean a TikTok dance for the past week.

～

April 8, 2020. As if things couldn't possibly get any worse, they did. Bernie dropped out of the democratic primary today. Which means I'm going to have to vote for Biden, all of this cannot be good for my mental health. Ryan is especially upset, he's been a hard Bernie supporter since 2015, he said he just wanted to able to vote for him once, even in a primary, even if he knew he wasn't going to win, and now he doesn't have that chance. Katie said she's not going to vote at all, when she said it I jumped on her, everyone in the group chat did, it's essential that we vote, even if we have to vote for Biden its better than not voting at all, but I understand where she's coming from, it feels hopeless, we all said we don't even want to have children if T*ump stays for another term. But we shouldn't have jumped on Katie, it's just as bad as not voting, we're all in this together.

I'm Skyping Ryan tonight, we haven't talked in a few days besides texting, we need something to distract ourselves from the Bernie news, we're going to watch Doctor Strange, plan on drinking quite a bit tonight after, I've been doing that recently, drinking, we all have actually, there's lots of jokes online, there's a sting of drink tutorials on TikTok and Twitter, it's a weird side effect of social distancing, were all unemployed and stressed as hell and liquor stores are some of the few stores still open so, were drinking.

～

April 12, 2020, Easter. Weirdest Easter to date. To have something to look forward to my family decided to do a small brunch, my mom made a vegetarian egg casserole, I made a vegan oatmeal bake and we got bagels, lox, spreads and lots of champagne and orange juice. I was home last year for Easter. I was planning on coming home from school this year for the weekend, we usually switch each year from my Mom's side of the family to my Dad's we were already planning on having a much smaller Easter than usual, we were going to my Grandparent's house and do the usual Easter diner, we still do an Easter egg hunt because we have a few little cousins in the family, soon it'll be my older cousins' kids were doing it for. My grandma always makes way too much Italian food, her way of reminding us we're not completely Irish. She is from Malta, grew up in Brooklyn, but my family consists of a bunch of blonde-haired blue-eyed men and my Grandpa's still got his Irish accent, so she reminds us were not completely Irish from her amazing chicken cutlets, stuffed shells, sausage and peppers, its watered down Italian but it's still amazing, thinking about it is making my mouth water. But we didn't have that this year, this year we had bagels lox and champagne from 12pm to 10pm because we finally had something to celebrate.

A few days ago, my parents and I started the garden in our backyard, something else to keep us busy especially once classes ended. There's no end in sight for any of this so it'll be me and the basil plants until further notice. I'm starting to get used to being home, the option of leaving is still missed but I've picked up guitar again, I'm slowly remembering how to play it's been a few years but I'm enjoying it, I think my dad is too, he's been desperate to get me or my sister to start playing an instrument again.

There's two more weeks ahead of me until finals week, I have a music video project draft and an environmental sustainability assignment due tomorrow, I was planning on doing them today, that did not happen, although there seems to be no end in sight the passing of time still shows me were closer to that end date than we were yesterday, whenever that end date may be.

April 14, 2020. Woke up around 10 a.m. today, I'm finding it less and less important to get up at a certain time, I know that'll catch up with me, a schedule is a very important way to stay sane. We had a FaceTime call with my grandmother this morning, she's in a hospice nursing home, last time I saw her was a few days before her home got locked down, my mom, sister, aunt, and I all stopped by for a few hours, this was well before anyone was wearing masks or staying home but they had us use hand sanitizer, asked us where we'd been in the last two weeks and took our temperature. We found out a few days ago two workers and a resident had tested positive, we expect its more, from what we've heard nursing homes have not been forthcoming with how far the virus has spread and we unfortunately don't expect much different from "The Manor" but we're just hoping the best for my grandma and were talking with her as often as we can. Not that there's anything to talk about, I told her I scheduled my classes for next semester at least three times, my mom went through every plant in our new garden, and I think my dad went through the particulars of his day by the half hour, and we still had 20 minutes of video call to fill. There's nothing to talk about, nothing new is happening accept the death toll is rising and more things are being closed. I really can't imagine how this is affecting everyone's mental health.

I've certainly gone a bit off the rails a few times now. I did a face mask last night, highlight of my week and I sent my boyfriend at least 20 snapchats of the process, this morning I danced to nothing while I made vegetables and eggs for breakfast for the 4th day in a row. Might as well be Groundhog Day, that might honestly be better than the progressive severity of everything. These journals are really helping me keep track of days and somewhat understand how I'm feeling, at least be aware of it, if not I might just forget what day it is all together. Every day seems to have that weird Sunday afternoon anxiety, even the weekends don't feel much different apart from drinking after 5 p.m. And I know there are plenty of people who have it much worse, I'm not a nurse or a doctor, everyone in my family is safe and healthy but that doesn't mean I'm not scared, overwhelmed, overstimulated by the news, the numbers being thrown at us just getting bigger and more unimaginable by the day, and I've stopped listening to the president altogether, the nonsense spewing out of him and his Twitter has nearly sent me to tears more than a few times, I am lucky to be living in New York, we're at the epicenter of the whole thing but at least Mayor De Blasio and Governor Cuomo are sane I seriously think they're doing the best they can and I am so grateful to be able to trust them rather than the bumbling idiot in the White House. . . .

Speaking of going of the rails . . . these journals may just devolve into therapy sessions with myself.

∿

April 15, 2020. We learned about the WWII Mass Observation journals that these COVID journals are based on in class today. It was jarring, unsettling, fascinating, I never could have imagined a few months ago that I would be in a time even remotely like WWII and here I am personally understanding a journal written by a girl in 1939. I found this project incredibly fascinating when I first started and the thought that one day my journal may be in a collection like the mass observation journals we're reading is unbelievable. I was writing some of these journals yesterday before reading the WWII journals for class and having everything so fresh and seeing all the similarities was incredibly unsettling and made this whole situation seem much bigger.

The WWII journals we read were written by a girl named Muriel Green, she was 18 in 1939 living in Norfolk. She mentions the depressiveness of businesses not being what they used to be, like all the stores closing at the beginning of the pandemic. She also writes about rationing, and as we're not rationing yet this is definitely a bit worse than we have it we are seeing echoes of that today, the shortages in supermarkets, the hesitation to even go to supermarkets. And I feel I have to keep reiterating, this is absolutely not as bad as the second world war, I'm not sure there are many things that could be worse than atrocities of the second world war but reading civilian journals, seeing the war from a far, it feels a lot like what we're going through now.

There was also a bit of the journals that discussed Muriel going to a meeting in the city. At this point civilians had been given gas masks in order to protect themselves from the tear gas that was constantly covering city streets. Muriel mentions that she and others were holding their gas masks but at the risk of seeming too over dramatic they were not putting them on, the gas subsided, and they continued on without them until she got to the meeting where they were hit with a room full of tear gas. No one had worn their gas masks as directed and because of this they all got hit with tear gas very badly, Muriel even writes "I suppose it was a case of feeling 'silly' to put one on when other people had not got theirs on" sounds eerily familiar doesn't it? Everyone dismissing face masks and gloves to avoid seeming overdramatic, until it was too late.

April 20, 2020. Nothing noteworthy has been going on recently. I've spent every day at home, I've stopped counting how many days we've been quarantined, it's over a month now. My sisters sneaking out tonight to a bonfire with Jonathan, she's wearing a mask and gloves. I'm not sure how much they're social distancing though.

I'm a bit nervous, I've stopped going to stores "just to get out" because it's not even enjoyable anymore, everyone's nervous, the lines are wrapped around blocks, not because everyone's getting to the stores but because they're only letting a few people in at a time and the people online have to wait six feet apart. Last time I went to a store was to get hair dye for Grace, we dyed and bleached her hair about a week ago, we went to Target first, forgetting about the lines and we showed up and couldn't understand what was going on but once we remembered we tried CVS, the line wasn't as long they were letting in only half capacity at a time, we got our hair dye and got the hell out. It's not fun outside anymore.

April 26, 2020. I gave myself a haircut this morning. I should've gotten one when I got home from school, I needed one desperately so I did it myself, checking off all the boxes on quarantine bingo this week, I've made at least five new kinds of cocktails this past weekend, I cut and bleached my hair, I've stayed in my house over 48 hours, it feel so incredibly normal now, I've completely stopped being aware how long we've been quarantined, it's been weeks since I've left my house past my backyard.

I have a week left of classes, finals start tomorrow I'm not sure what life's going to look like when I have no classes, my mom said me and my sister might be able to start working with her again at her job, we'd be going in to help clear out the office since they paid out their lease while no one's been going in. Anything is better than the alternative of completely unscheduled days for an undetermined amount of time, no amount of arts and crafts could fill up that many days.

I'm too old to get blamed for everything . . .

April 2, 2020

Mad Millennial

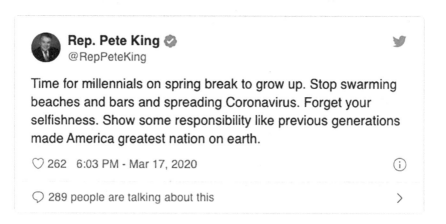

> **Rep. Pete King** ✔
> @RepPeteKing
>
> Time for millennials on spring break to grow up. Stop swarming beaches and bars and spreading Coronavirus. Forget your selfishness. Show some responsibility like previous generations made America greatest nation on earth.
>
> ♡ 262   6:03 PM - Mar 17, 2020   ⓘ
>
> ◯ 289 people are talking about this   ⟩

It's always felt like a cool thing to dump on young people and blame them for everything. But something that really grinds the gears of those of us in the Millennial generation is when we get blamed for things that aren't our fault.

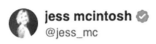

jess mcintosh ✔
@jess_mc

I need everyone on the news to stop blaming Millennials on spring break. That is Gen Z.

Millennials are home trying to keep their children out of the frame on zoom while they work.

♡ 6,331   11:38 AM - Mar 20, 2020   ⓘ

💬 869 people are talking about this   ＞

Basically, if anyone wants to dump on young people, the headline has to read millennial. Watch what you say Boomer, or I won't teach you how to unmute yourself on Zoom.

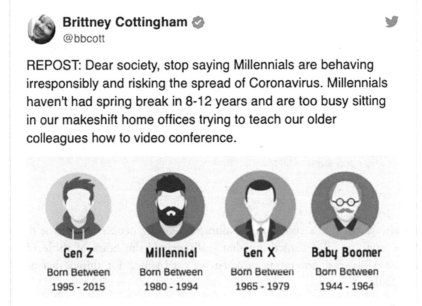

Brittney Cottingham ✔
@bbcott

REPOST: Dear society, stop saying Millennials are behaving irresponsibly and risking the spread of Coronavirus. Millennials haven't had spring break in 8-12 years and are too busy sitting in our makeshift home offices trying to teach our older colleagues how to video conference.

Gen Z	Millennial	Gen X	Baby Boomer
Born Between 1995 - 2015	Born Between 1980 - 1994	Born Between 1965 - 1979	Born Between 1944 - 1964

♡ 139   10:15 AM - Mar 23, 2020   ⓘ

💬 77 people are talking about this   ＞

Food for Thought

April 2, 2020

ANN TRAITOR

We went food shopping today, after being home for nearly two weeks.

To be honest, we were scared. The stories we heard from our cashier neighbor—frightening in the extreme! Long lines; people waiting for an hour or more to get in; people not finding what they needed and getting frustrated and angry; the shock of empty shelves; people stealing items out of other people's carts—none of this gave us any confidence at all. Based on all of this, my daughter and I decided to go together to make it quicker and to go really late in the evening, at an off-peak time.

It was surreal. There were a good number of people in the store but that was not the most surprising part: it was the silence. There was no background "music-to-shop-by," no announcements on "sale items fresh from the bakery," no "people-out-and-about" noise of any kind. The only thing we heard was the muffled shuffle of feet. Even the creaky carts were silent. No one chatted or even said "excuse me." Wide-eyed and fearful, people pushed their carts, looked at everyone else as a potential food-stealing enemy, and grabbed things quickly off shelves. One woman was actively crying, tears streaming down her face, as she pushed her mostly empty cart from one aisle to another. She made not a sound.

We call him "COVID warrior"

April 2, 2020

MICHELLE HENDLEY

In response to the coronavirus pandemic, one of my many cousins set up a WhatsApp chat group for our family so that we can stay in touch during this time. I have at least 25 first cousins on my father's side of the family, most of whom are on the chat group. Many of my cousins are parents and grandparents. The family is very large and scattered across the world: Jamaica, the country where my cousins, grandparents, parents, aunts, uncles, siblings, and I were born, Canada, Australia, the United Kingdom, and the United States. The U.S.-based family lives in New York (me), Virginia, Florida, California, and Texas. It is a lively, multi-generational, diverse, and widely dispersed group which makes for spirited chat.

The initial messages on the chat that I saw consisted of family members joyously greeting each other and expressing their gratitude for this platform on which to communicate. Tidings of staying healthy and staying at home were exchanged. Pictures of family, flowers, food, mountains, and beaches were posted; however, there was one post that defied the jocular chat exchange. Bobbie, my cousin Geoffrey's wife, posted that he was out of bed and on the couch, the worst was over and that he was recovering. Geoffrey lives in Texas, works in the medical field, and travels a lot for his job. He is a husband, father, grandfather, brother, and cousin. He is also one of the over 200,000 confirmed U.S. COVID-19 cases.

Thankfully, Geoffrey recovered from COVID-19. My cousin Barbie asked Geoffrey to share the symptoms of his illness with the family chat group so that we would know what to expect in the event that one of us became infected with the coronavirus. Geoffrey generously shared his battle with the disease. His illness was a real wake-up call for the rest of us. It was dreadful. It was miserable. He had a fever for 12 days. He had no energy. He had no appetite. I thought that some good could come from Geoffrey's suffering by sharing it with others. Geoffrey generously agreed that I could share his symptoms on the pandemic diary project. I am grateful for his willingness to share his account with us because it vividly illustrates the seriousness of the disease:

> . . . at first, I felt tired with just a little lack of energy. Fever and decline came on quickly. Next day the dry cough started and lack of appetite. Energy level dropped to very low and stayed that way for two weeks. Overall feeling of bad illness like you would feel having a bad case of the flu. Although from a subjective point of view it felt different than anything I had felt before. The expected aches and pains associated with fever and staying in bed for so long. Some of the main symptoms I did not experience are tightening in the chest and shortness of breath. I took shallow breaths to avoid stimulating the cough as much as I could. I pray none of you have to experience this and I feel blessed I did not get to the point of hospitalization.

This illness was so bad, my cousin used a very expressive, colorful, Jamaican curse-word to describe it. I won't write it here because only Jamaicans would understand the meaning and forcefulness of the word. And it's not a nice word although, trust me, it is an apt description. Any illness that gives you a fever for 12 days deserves to be cursed at.

Geoffrey recently received the all clear from the health department. He is released from quarantine. His wife Bobbie is in quarantine until the middle of April. His daughter and family will be in quarantine until early April. He may have antibodies now to protect him from another bought of COVID-19; however, he is taking no chances. He continues to practice social distancing because he does "not want to tangle with COVID-[curse word] ever again!" Geoffrey is wise. He knows firsthand the power of COVID-19. He is a survivor. He is resilient. He is grateful. One of my other cousins paid tribute to Geoffrey by nicknaming him "COVID Warrior." He is a warrior. He is my family's COVID-19 warrior.

Thank you Cosima

April 3, 2020

Darren D. Chase

Some dogs wear bandanas and make it look good. These dogs are born to it—endowed with a confident, frisky, cool spirit that finds expression jauntily wearing a bandana. Cosima is a bandana dog.

With recent advice encouraging the wearing of face masks in public, Cosima's bandana wardrobe is being repurposed. Thank you, Cosima, for your sweetness and love, and thank you for the face masks.

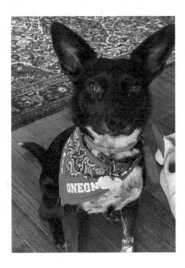 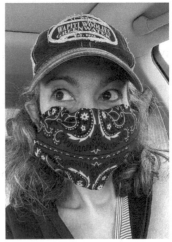

Diary Entries

April 4, 2020

JULIAN GOTIANGCO

April 4

Dear Diary,

I woke up feeling sick. The sickest I have been in a long time, and I didn't even realize it. I had chills the whole morning, and my mom checked my temperature and saw I had a fever. I had to go to the hospital. Thankfully, within a day or two, I got better. I did not have the dreaded virus. I'm just happy I'm healthy and safe at home with my family.

April 8

Well, here's some good news. I got an opportunity to do some acting during this time of distance learning. My friend Stephen is a senior student, and he is studying theater. He is taking a directing class, and he asked me if I wanted to be in a short 2–3 minute scene. We would have only a few only rehearsals through Zoom and then record the final performance. I felt honored that he thought of me. So, I accepted the opportunity. I am not going to be on a big stage, but just to be able to act again makes me happy—even if it is a short scene. Rehearsals start next week.

April 12

Happy Easter! It feels strange to be at home for Easter because I usually visit family. I miss all my aunts, uncles, and cousins, and I just wonder every day how they are holding up during all of this. My mom made roasted chicken for dinner and my sister helped her make pumpkin pie for dessert. It was a great meal, yet I wished we were at a larger gathering.

April 13

I'm not sure what number week we are up to in distance learning, and I am too lazy to check my previous diary entries to find the answer. I was a little sad today because this week would have been tech week for Once Upon a Mattress. Tech week rehearsals are the last few rehearsals before opening night and the cast would get to wear costumes and mics. I wish I was at school with my friends getting ready for the show, but it was for the best that we were asked to stay home. I still talk to my friends and check up on them. I think it's very important to do that in a time like this.

April 15

Today would have been opening night for Once Upon a Mattress. I wish we could have been at school today and put on our show. I really miss all my friends.

April 19

I feel like I should read more books, but I have not made time to do that. I decided to read The Martian by Andy Weir. I saw the movie version with Matt Damon, and I thought that movie was great. It had a very pro-science message, and I just loved the creativity Matt Damon's character had in order to survive on Mars. Also, he found himself facing adversity, but his optimism never wavered. I think this is very inspiring and something we should all try to aspire to especially considering what's going on in the world with the Coronavirus. Anyways, I hear the book is better than the movie. I am hoping to finish the book by June. Wish me luck!

April 27

Today I finished rehearsals for Stephen's directing assignment. I was very happy how the scene turned out. I had so much fun helping Stephen with his assignment. It reminded me of how much I missed performing and theater in general.

April 28

Today is the last day of classes. All I need to do is take my finals. I hope they go well. This will be my last entry. I miss my friends. I miss being at school. I miss giving my parents hugs. I miss eating out. I miss going out to the movie theater. There are so many things I miss. I hope that this virus will pass soon.

Envision . . . Predict . . . Imagine

April 6, 2020

VICTORIA CHICOLO

Imagine we knew that this would happen? If we were able to predict it . . . Would we have been able to prevent it? To stop all the chaos? Or would it still have spread so fast . . . so uncontrollably?

Imagine someone in the past saw the future. Saw this massive chaos without even knowing? Did someone in the world have a dream . . . or even vision . . . of the world shutting down? . . . Did the world shut down?

Imagine if life doesn't get back to normal? Is this life the new normal?

Imagine someone in the world sees the future . . . dreams of what it will be? Does someone in the world know if life will get better . . . or even worse?

Imagine someone in the world knows the outcome of each route. Would they tell anyone? Would anyone believe them? Do they even believe what they envision?

Imagine if you were able to know the future . . . Know what will become of the world after this chaos is over . . . Would you want to know . . . or are you better just imagining?

April 2020
April 8, 2020

DANIELLE D.

April 8, 2020

This quarantine is driving me absolutely nuts! I feel like I have literally been thrown into isolation. I want to point out that I am writing this part at 5:18am on a sad Friday morning (I can't sleep).

My day-to-day now consists of waking up at the grand hour of 2pm. Yup, every day. To be more exact I have been waking up at around 1:49pm which I think is weird. A coincidence maybe? Okay, so next I will just lay in bed on my laptop checking blackboard, just barely making deadlines for all the work I have. Then next I will emerge myself into the world of video games or sit down with a snack and watch a movie. In all situations I am home, in my room, sitting on my bed, all alone. But am I alone? Not really because I've got my family . . . and my dog. My point is this whole no contact with the outside world is so mentally constraining and depriving for my young developing mind. I am a growing individual here! Okay, maybe I am a little aggressive, but I just really believe that's an important issue that could come about after this. Having people have no contact with others could literally turn them nuts.

I am just going to say that all jokes aside, this pandemic is the scariest thing in my current life span.

April 10, 2020

I am so tired of sitting around all day and pretending like it's okay. This pandemic is so stupid. Let me just say the people who go around honking their horns and yelling "Happy Birthday" at some houses are really, really annoying. It is adorable and nice, but not when you get stuck in the middle of it on your way home from getting the essential toilet paper that's always out of stock. Also, my neighbors were trying to leave their homes and these stupid cars blocked their way out.

I have been eating a lot of McDonalds recently and that has not made me very happy.

Don't get me wrong, I love some good chicken nuggets, but every day? No.

April 11, 2020

My parents are super worried about this pandemic. They are older people in their late fifties early sixties so they should have worry. This virus is affecting a great number of the older population. My father was a NYC fireman at Squad 41 in the Bronx for 26 years. He went through 9/11 and had first-hand experiences of true, raw trauma and tragedy. He had compromised lungs because of this. He is at high risk to get this virus and that scares me. He's my dad, if he's not around then I'm not sure what to do or how my household would stay functioning. I would hate to see him survive one tragedy but not live through another. I have seen other first responders during 9/11 dying from this virus. I just want this to be over, no more scaring us.

April 16, 2020

COVID-19 was thought to have been started because people were eating bats in China.

It's weird but I've learned in my life that it is better not to judge. Anyway, recently they found out something so crazy about the real cause. I'm not one to keep up with the news so I'm not exactly sure on all the details, but apparently it was started in a lab and China was testing it.

They were apparently testing it to use as a possible weapon to bring everyone else's economy down and have their economy go up. And I heard the spread was because someone in the lab passed it to their girlfriend and then it spread. This is one crazy story. I am not sure how true this is, but I do, however, know that it did not come from eating bats and it came from a lab.

It is crazy to think that a China was creating this to utilize it as a weapon against the world. A pandemic happens every 100 years but this one could have been avoided. Although they do say history repeats itself.

I hope I'm safe from this and I hope I come out better. I hope my morals aren't so messed up like the people testing a deadly disease and letting it spread.

April 19, 2020

I have been waking up recently at 4pm and going to sleep somewhere between 5am and 9am every day. This is driving me crazy. I waste my days and spend my nights doing just about nothing. I do try and utilize that time by doing homework . . . sometimes.

So far with my workload I have nearly finished everything. I am done with one class completely and almost done with two others. This is so exciting as it means that the end is near.

Summer is coming! Although I would have liked my freshman year as a student at SUNY Oneonta to end differently, I am grateful for the experiences I went through and the time I spent on campus. I will never forget my freshman year. It was full of so much drama and fun that it is impossible to ever forget. It can easily be said that it is the best and worst year of my life.

I miss campus a lot. Walking around every day on campus was so much fun. I lived in Golding Hall which was the absolute best freshman dorm on campus. It was the newest dorm building and I was lucky enough to be in it. I had all my friends in the building, and everything was great.

I even had a single room because my roommate and I got in a fight. I am not going to get into that, but just know she made my life absolutely miserable. She was one reason why it was the worst year ever. But her moving out was the best thing to ever happen as I never got a new roommate and I lived on my own for half a semester. I did not have to worry about anyone but myself and that was an amazing feeling. I miss that a lot. I miss walking down that hallway and being happy going to my friends' room down the hall. So serene. I also miss doing things outside of campus with my friends. The parties are truly missed during this time of isolation.

April 24, 2020

My favorite thing to do is be by myself during this time. There is nothing like peace and quiet. But that is hard to get when you live in a home with five other people and the house is about two feet big. I just wish I could be in my dorm room right now listening to music and doing my homework. That is really peaceful. I mean, I do that now, but it isn't the same.

Oneonta is truly one of my favorite places to be. It is where all my friends are and where my future is. I miss it so much. Everything about it I miss. I just wish I could go back in time to the beginning of the spring semester and cherish those moments again. At this rate of the virus, we do not even know if we will be going back to school, but I will hope.

April 28, 2020

This is my last day writing. I want to say that I enjoyed journaling my days over this short period of time. It gave me time to reflect on what I was doing and thinking. This semester has been a wild ride. I met a ton of new people, learned how to snowboard, improved my grades, and learned so much about myself. This whole quarantine experience will stay with me for the rest of my life. I may just keep journaling because I want to look back on this and remember what I went through. I hope I will get good grades during this time and achieve the best I could despite the circumstances.

My favorite part of this experience was getting to spend time with myself. I am finding self-love and am actively caring for myself better. I also have been working on my compassion skills with my family as we haven't always had the greatest relationships. I will not miss quarantine, but I am surprisingly glad it happened, and I will continue to thrive during this time.

Thank you for reading.

Diary Entry

April 10, 2020

Britney DeCoster

I feel like a mouse in a trap. I'm stuck here with no idea what is going on. The virus is spiking in NY. My mom works at a nursing home where most, if not all, of the patients have tested positive and now she doesn't feel well. I just wish this monster would go away just as fast as it spread. It has made me pessimistic about everything. The government can say whatever they want about it but no one really knows what to do. Worst case scenario, it's like the Walking Dead (hopefully without the zombies), rationing food and supplies. I've already started eating less just in case the supermarkets and public businesses are shut down.

As terrible as this plague has been I've realized that I am very lucky. I have my family that loves me, I have food, I have a place to rest my head. There are people other there of all ages that needed the free lunch system at schools to eat daily. There are people that depend heavily on food pantries. There are people in abusive households that have been stuck there for weeks now. There are people who don't have access to their medicine. There are people who can't even hide from the monster because they don't have a home.

Yes, families fight all the time but at least we are all together during this time.

I'm Falling Down On My Ethnographic Responsibilities and I Need To Be OK With That

April 10, 2020

SALLIE HAN

To be honest, I've felt both like I have an ethnographer's responsibility to document this time—and also so overwhelmed with just holding it together (with teaching, with my people at home, with all of the feelings . . .) that I get a little cranky and resentful about feeling this imperative to be meaningfully productive with this moment. I AM ALREADY A FULL-TIME PROFESSOR, PARENT, AND SPOUSE. So, like, I'm not baking sourdough or sewing masks—much less collecting data on, say, experiences of pregnant women during COVID isolation. I don't even wish I were someone who could do it all. Right now, I just wish the sun was shining in Oneonta, but it's Friday, April 10, and it's snowing.

I miss my friends.

April 10, 2020

JULIA HARKINS

I really do. I was a sophomore in college this year and feel like I lost so many memories that should have happened up at school. I sit in my house and hear from almost no one, which is a huge reality check. As young as I am, I am a part of the compromised. I am a severe asthmatic.

I wish there was more I could do to help myself and others during this isolation. But I can't.

Hopefully, this will be over soon.

Impulse Spending

April 10, 2020

SIERRA AUTUMN GOLD

As if I thought my online shopping addiction
Began and ended while physically attending college,
it snuck up on me, its virulent fangs piercing my wallet
"buy the Xbox" it whispered, devilishly into my ear
here I am, days later, up late, playing games
one Xbox "richer"

Learning

April 10, 2020

Lexi Veitch

Classes have moved to a digital format and my childhood bedroom has suddenly taken the place of a library, dorm room, gym, etc. I am learning to live, work and play in a confined space while trying to stay connected with friends and family. I have noticed my productivity comes in waves. This time requires that we be patient with ourselves. The days feel as if they are melting together. My mom and I have been able to practice our cooking and baking skills and we are starting to experiment with new recipes. Long walks on the local bike path have been the highlight of my days. I have picked up trash along the roads near my house and have seen other citizens doing the same. While people are consuming less and commuting less, Earth is receiving a much-needed rest.

Prof. Sal Diary

April 10, 2020

Prof. Salvatore Salvaggio

12:36 pm. It's Snowing. Cat's sleeping. Slippers off. If we can take this isolation being enclosed, I am pretty sure the trip to Mars my grandkids might take is a possibility. I hope the puzzles we ordered come in the mail today. Milk is running low.

Pretty Sick Time to Be Alive

April 10, 2020

CAROL BEAN

This is a pretty sick time to be alive.

It's pretty sick that we are living through a historic pandemic.

It's pretty sick that seniors lost precious time.

Sick that the death toll is increasing each day, that people are not staying inside, that we cannot hug our loved ones.

It's pretty sick that air pollution is decreasing, that people are coming together to support each other, that we get to step back and hug ourselves.

Breathe in the air, but not too much because it's a pretty sick time to be alive.

Fitness and Quarantine

April 10, 2020

CORDELL ABERNATHY

Rose late today at 7 am. Leaped onto my elliptical for 5 hours and a 35-minute strength training session with the Vengeance Strength Kvlt bros. Rainy and cold or else I would walk outside during the COVID outbreak. With all gyms closed, I rely on my fitness know-how and body weight to make do until they open again.

Chores with my mum pass the time along with homework to get done before the weekend. Easter is still happening for my family, and we are all together. I'm wicked happy and blessed everyone is safe and healthy in my family. Hail to the Sun to keep all men safe during this trying time.

Death Is Death

April 11, 2020

Naomi Graham

On April 4th, my mother-in-law passed away. She was a gentle and loving, supportive woman, not at all like the stereotype of a dreadful interfering mother-in-law that you see in films and commercials. She was living with dementia in a local nursing home, and as she declined, my husband and I would go try to peek in the windows to see her, as we were not allowed inside. Finally, when they realized it was the end of life, they let us inside, and we spent the last 3 days sitting by her side, reading poems, singing, reading from the bible, weeping, and holding her hand. So, I am very grateful that we got to spend that time with her, and my heart goes out to the many folks whose loved ones are passing in hospitals without the sound of a loved voice or the touch of a loved hand.

But then the other thing, the part that makes this COVID diary worthy or weird, is that she did not pass away from COVID-19. And I feel I have to say that to everyone I tell. "My mother-in-law passed away, but it was not from COVID-19," so they won't think that she was infected, that I am infected, that we are under the shadow, this dreadful, all-powerful raptor that has spread out its vast dark wings above us all, our county, our state, our country, our world. It was just death. Like life and death. The mortality that infects us all.

Uncertain Times

April 11, 2020

Janice Hambor

In uncertain times, imagination can be a blessing and a curse. I am torn between checking the news to stay informed and boycotting the media to keep negative and paranoid thoughts at bay. In truth, it is impossible to distinguish between what is realistic and what is paranoid. How much of what we hear is an attempt by those in power to control the masses? And to what end? Some stories seem to lean toward producing mass hysteria; others to negate the extent to which this pandemic is crippling every system in society. I don't know what to believe. I am afraid I am taking this too seriously. I am terrified that I am not. It is the uncertainty, the isolation, and the powerlessness that feeds my fear.

Now more than ever, I must channel my faith. I tell myself that nothing is ever certain. That despite the seemingly overwhelming circumstances around me, God's got this. Though I haven't faced anything like this before, I have lived through some perilous times. I hope. I pray. I will not allow fear to dominate me.

We are in this together. God bless us.

Desolate

April 11, 2020

Nadia Boyea

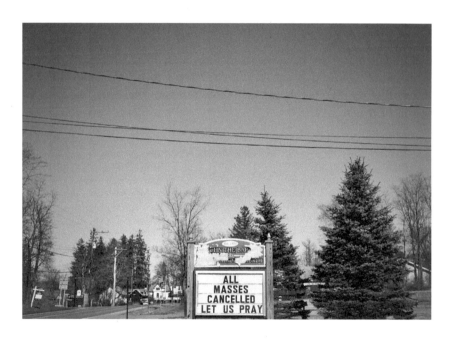

The experience of social distancing and self-quarantines has taken a toll on everyone I know in one way or another. Graduations are cancelled or postponed. New mothers can't show off their newborn babies to friends and family. Kids and their parents are stuck at home; seeing them playing outside while I walk by knowing it is their only reprieve is sad. There's a small park one house away from mine that is usually crawling with the neighborhood kids with the start of the warmer weather, and now it's rare that anyone is there at all. There's only so much we can do, and that is to actively do nothing. I've personally found this to be a really stressful time, knowing I really don't have the option to go see friends, even though everyone was forced home from college.

The religious community is very prevalent in my town, this is one of three within a two-mile radius that has canceled services.

There are now 37 cases in my county, and I think it has just started to be taken seriously. Being as far upstate as we are, there was a lot of ignorance thinking that the virus would not reach us, but alas, those escaping the diseased city sought safety in their summer homes and without knowing it brought the virus with them. There was the initial panic buying, and the grocery store remains busier than it probably should be. As of now, there are about a dozen people I know of who have either been tested, gone to the emergency room, had to self-quarantine due to exposure, and one has even died.

Local businesses have been suffering, most food places have temporarily closed. Those that remain open still seem to have customers as I've driven by, but everyone is so wary of each other. The virus has made us fearful of living.

Hollowness

April 13, 2020

Kim Se-Chan

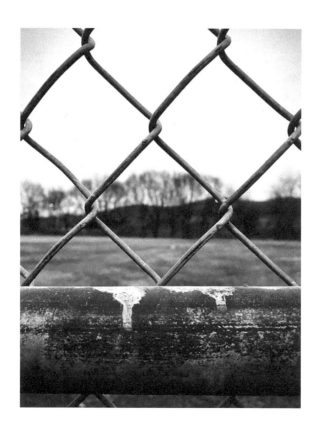

Ever since the extended spring break, everything had changed. I mean everything. There were no longer Friday gatherings, no longer 'classes' and no longer freedom.

I have come to Oneonta as an exchange student for one semester. I don't regret it by the way. If I had to come again, I would definitely choose SUNY Oneonta, no second thought. It was mostly the people that I liked. The kind and funny professors who helped me get through this new studying environment. The friends I made and encountered, none of them were unfriendly or unkind. Actually, they were so nice that it encouraged me to be a better person.

Now, thinking that those people have left. There is so much hollowness in my heart.

These times are not for people with anxiety!

April 13, 2020

Cindi Hall

I have anxiety and my heart races just with thoughts of dreaded things that are upcoming. I am older and this just started recently in the past 3 years because of many things in my life that are just not controllable. I have always been a "fixer" and I cannot "fix" what is going on around me today; this causes me sleepless nights and crying jags. The one thing that keeps going through my mind with all this chaos is, "Will the world ever be normal again?"

I.e.—Will we want to wear masks for a long time after this is done because we don't trust officials to judge if it is safe? Will the job market recover? Is this the next Depression? How many will die? Will family or friends that I know die from this? If many people get sick in this rural area, how will we have enough ventilators? Will I die from this? These thoughts have caused me to update my obituary and death instructions and tell my family where they are located. I am not afraid of dying but I would like to stick around to see my grandchildren grow up. I also worry about my brother and daughter in law who work in healthcare. My Mom is in a nursing home with dementia and Parkinson's, will this take her life? If she does get COVID-19, will I be allowed to see her in her final hours? I haven't seen her since March 6th because of the lockdown at her facility. She doesn't understand any of this and thinks we just left her there to die. She is angry and lashing out at the nurses and aides. I don't want her to die with that frame of mind, in turmoil.

We moved in with my mother-in-law a year ago and she has dementia also. She is very confused and is shocked by the death tolls every day but she only understands that no one can find toilet paper at the store. It is funny the way the mind protects people from evil in this world. I asked our Pastor to FaceTime with her today because when he prays with her it seems to give her peace. What will give me peace though?

April Showers bring . . . a boatload of work!
April 13, 2020

CORDELL ABERNATHY

Morning spent working out on the home elliptical. Shelter in place = no gym = no friends = no chuckles and jeers. I completed by 4 hr. cardio sesh and 100 pushups, 100 crunches, and 100 . . . no wait . . . only 60 kettle-bell swings. I don't want to be a weakling goober! Better luck tomorrow.

Rain Rain go away!! No walk outside today! 66 degrees but rain all day. My goal for the week: Complete a 10-page essay for African American art due in May, start and finish making the garden tidy from last year i.e., tilling the soil, transplanting worms to make the soil healthier, and de-weeding it, and working on at least 1 creative venture. Listened to my dungeon-synth project today and realized that along with getting my body back to "model perfect" as it was in 2018, I also need to work on getting my keyboard harmonies up to snuff . . . good things DO NOT happen to those who wait too long!

Not seeing my partner of 9 years is wicked sad and gives me hard-core anxiety, but we call daily and Skype, and I have 2 of my besties from Rick Owens who call me daily just to shoot the breeze and talk fashion. Apparently "apocalyptic chic" is out and "Malibu Barbie/island girl" is in. Go figure, eh? Well, I started my 10-page research paper, typing it all out as I write it by hand before, so my thoughts don't scatter. I HIGHLY recommend this technique for those who are diagnosed with ADHD/OCD/Anxiety (like I have) as it helps your thoughts stay contained and focused. I accomplished 3/4 assignments for CGP today, so I suppose I'm "ahead of things." Cleaned the entire house top to bottom, managed to stick to the "Karl Lagerfeld diet" (I highly recommend this diet to anyone looking to get "bikini ready" in the midst of quarantine). No quarantine 15 for this boi!

Building a wardrobe for myself that is both comfortable and trendy (even though no one but me, my folks, and Ithaca farmer's market people see me on the weekends) has helped me cope A LOT. Jeremy Scott, Wunderkind, and Kenzo/Roulon Smith have become my best friends. Nature walks and the Ithaca Farmers' market on Saturday have been my saving grace.

Hail to the Sun to keep shining His rays upon all who are worthy to receive them! Hael og Sael! Over and out . . .

Happiness

April 14, 2020

Kim Se-Chan

Whether you wanted it or not we've definitely been thinking about happiness a lot over a couple of weeks. What makes us happy? Becoming a CEO at a big corporation, having a thick wallet full of cash, getting straight A's, finding the love your life . . . Well, let's just start with petting your dog.

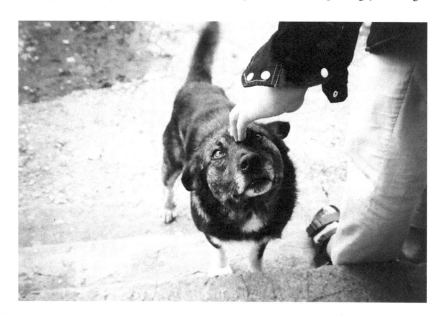

COVID-19 in 2020

April 14, 2020

GABRIELLE BUSH

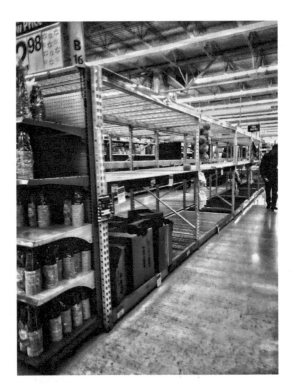

The public are panic buying toilet paper?

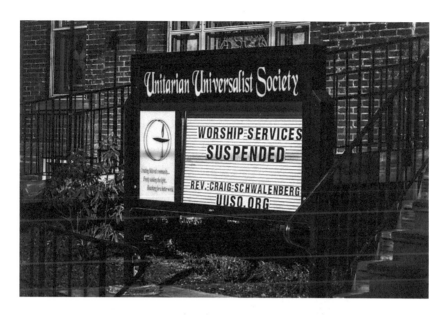

The places we normally go are empty and abandoned.

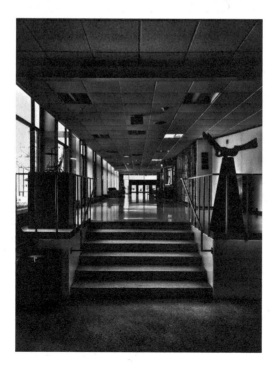

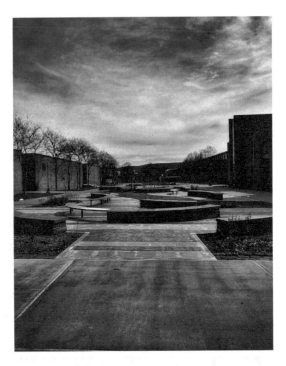

Meanwhile it seems as though people are making the time to get outside and enjoy nature, an escape from the quarantine. Other animals are blissfully ignorant to the social distancing rule.

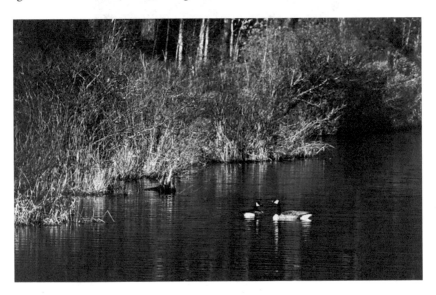

Students are stuck with an overwhelming amount of online course work finding it difficult to take breaks and remove themselves from it.

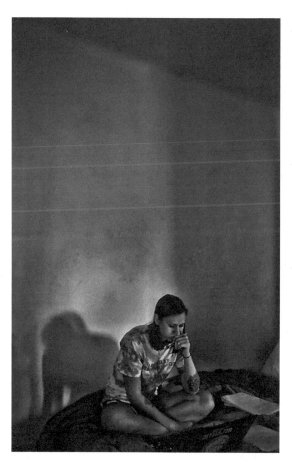

Hold out hope

April 14, 2020

Jillian Martelle

I can't believe that this is how we all have to start off 2020. This was supposed to be such an amazing year. It's the start of a new decade, but instead of thinking of all of the fun things that this year will bring I am just focused on making it through this hard time and hoping that this pandemic doesn't last too long. My life—like so many other people has been turned upside down. This is a time when people should be coming together, but instead, the entire world is shutting themselves inside their houses and locking their doors. When this whole situation first started, I was terrified. I worry all the time, and this was just another thing on a long list of things that swirl around in my head. When things started to get more serious my thoughts became more destructive. I started to really feel scared and unsafe. I didn't think that there was anywhere that I could go where I would be safe. How would I know if the virus could get to me or worse to my family? How do you protect the people that you love from something that you can't even see? As the entire world scrambles to make sense of this situation all I want is clarity and a concrete answer, but of course, this isn't something that I can get. We all just have to have hope. We have to hope that all of the hard work of the doctors, nurses, leaders, and even the work of everyday people will help to bring us out of this on the other side. Our world has never faced a situation like this. After spending so much of my time worrying about how this would end and what would change because of it I finally told myself that I had to stop. There is no point in worrying for the future when we don't focus on the present. We will all get through this. There will be sad times and losses, but there will also be courage and strength. In a time like this, no one is alone even if it feels that way. We are all going through this together and we will all come out stronger because of it. We just have to have hope.

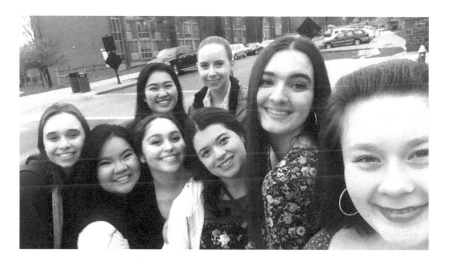

Here's to hoping for so many more adventures with these amazing people who have quickly become my second family!

Untouchable

April 14, 2020

Casey Collette

At first, I thought the media was being overdramatic. I didn't understand how a virus in China would affect my family and schooling in the United States.

When the virus was spreading to Italy and other countries, I thought I was untouchable. The United States knows what to do in a crisis, everything would be fine. We will take precautions before it even steps foot in America. There's nothing to worry about, I kept telling myself.

At the start of March, I thought that I was immune to this and was saddened to have to leave Oneonta. My family took me the week after spring break to get my stuff and I ended up staying a few days just to say goodbye to my home away from home.

I really thought we were going to come back to Oneonta at the end of March and this hysteria would be over. Little did I know this was the beginning of the end.

March 31st, 2020, my grandmother tested positive for COVID-19. The virus would then spread and infect my entire household.

During the time I was in Oneonta, my great-grandfather would be admitted into the hospital for shortness of breath. Turned out it was his congestive heart failure but once he was out of the hospital, he was too weak to care for himself anymore, so my family had to make the difficult decision to have my great-grandparents (92 & 94 years old) come live with us during this hard time. We have a multi-family house so we thought it was the best decision since there would be people to care for him here.

However, we began to see just how dangerous and real this virus was after this week. We all tried our best to be quarantined and stay clean. But my great-grandmother was the first one to show symptoms. She slowly got exhausted and started to have a high fever and bad cough. We called the emergency hotline provided by the state to make an appointment and they said to take her to a walk-in clinic.

My grandmother and great-grandmother took the test for the virus, but it would take 48 hours to hear the results. From that moment the walk-in doctor knew something was wrong and called an ambulance for my great-grandmother. She was rushed to the hospital because the virus is affecting her heart.

April 1st, the day after my grandmother's results came back positive, my great-grandmother's results came back positive as well.

My great-grandmother is still in the hospital being quarantined there while everyone in our house has been showing symptoms. It has been a roller coaster of emotions. How could something I thought was so far away affect my life this much?

My Sociological lens

April 14, 2020

Ho Hon Leung

While I am practicing social distancing well, I do take advantage of the quietness outside home. I walk around with my sociological eyes and observe how people fight against and cope with the outbreak. Work together in isolation. I see ourselves through my lens.

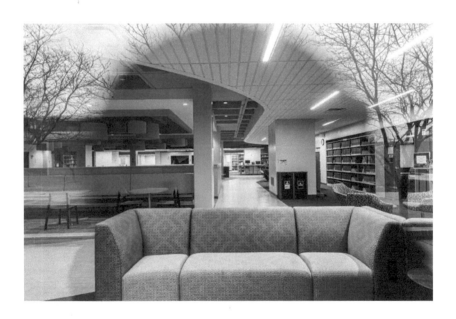

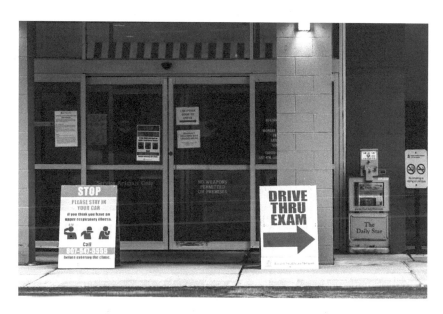

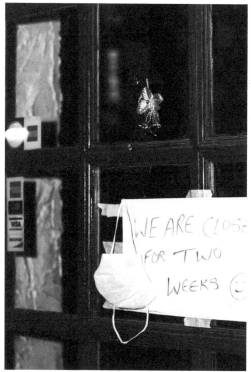

Everything Is Gonna be Groovy

April 14, 2020

Cordelle Abernathy

Worry and fear, two constant emotions for man, but through it all, Everything is gonna be groovy. War and disease occur but that's Nature's cycle, ya dig? This is another turn in the Wheel and a new age in the Kali Yugic cycle, but everything is still gonna be groovy. As long as we stay healthy, fit, smart, productive, and beautiful, it's all gonna be groovy.

But there will always be naysayers, negative neds and hypochondriacs, heads congested with the words of the media and not of their own judgment. Block it out, ya dig? Enjoy family and nature. Because after this ends and the world purifies itself, it's all gonna be groovy.

Frozen

April 14, 2020

Franklyn Macario

Everything seems to be Frozen. Our social lives, school, work, roads, parks, and the world in general. Everything is Frozen.

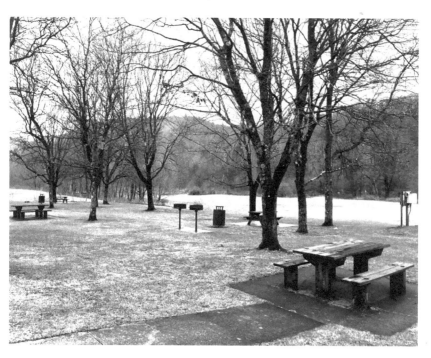

Craving Spring

April 15, 2020

LEXI VEITCH

Every year, at the end of a long winter, I crave for the blooming of flowers and the return of birds to fill the air with songs. Spring is coming, but it feels as if it is crawling to the start line. Spring brings new beginnings and thoughts of rejoicing with friends and family at picnics or baseball games. But as I think about everything that should be happening, I am reminded about what is yet to come. Uncertainty plagues our consciousness. We are living each day, preparing ourselves for bad news and hoping for the opposite. I am hanging on to the hope that in the unpredictability of the present, Spring remains on the horizon. A new day, that feels different than our yesterdays, will be here soon.

Easter

April 15, 2020

COURTNEY JONES

Things looked a little different this year.

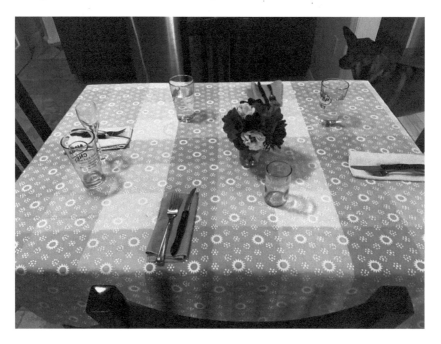

Isolated Fibromyalgia

April 15, 2020

GABRIELLE BUSH

I had a routine. One that started to work, and I could manage.

Although now everything has changed. My stress levels are high, routine is gone, and my pain has gotten worse. Living with Fibromyalgia during this time of isolation is hard. Online classes have caused more stress, irregular sleep patterns, limited amount of movements, irregular eating times. All of which can make the pain worse. I sit for hours on my laptop doing work and then I can't move because my body is stiff. Or I get out and take the dogs for a walk to take a break and I pay for it later in tears.

I feel myself breaking down.

As we near the end of the semester, my motivation for doing assignments gets lower and lower. I wake up in pain and I don't move from my bed, because I don't have to. I can work from there. Then my fiancé comes in with a cup of coffee, helps me into the shower, and I start my day. We do what we have to during these difficult situations, there are good days and bad.

Routines are important, and this change has negatively affected students in ways that many can't even imagine.

But we adapt, we survive and we overcome.

What will my kids remember about this time?

April 17, 2020

Sallie Han

My mother has accused me of thinking my children are pretty perfect. It isn't that exactly, though I'd admit I'm rather a doting parent ☺. It's like a prayer I say every night: As I settle down to sleep, I tell my husband that I love him and then I say aloud, ". . . and I love our two babies, too." Lately, because I want the last utterance, I make to be a little bit of a laugh, I add: "If we have to live through a global pandemic emergency, I'm glad it's with the three of you." He obligatorily harumphs and then I feel I can go to sleep. It isn't that I think my children are perfect, but I certainly think the world of them, by which I mean they're my world.

Yesterday, a friend asked me how my kids are doing at this time. At risk of confirming my mother's accusation, I will say that they have been pretty great during this past month at home. I have two babies, as I mentioned, and my 16-year-old is a 10th grader now home for the rest of the spring from boarding school, and my 12-year-old is a 7th grader at our local middle school. I feel bad about what my 16-year-old is missing. She was supposed to go to France for two weeks! and go "on tour" with her high school dance company! and so many other lovely plans that just have to wait now. Ditto my 12-year-old, who was having a terrific year at school, hitting his stride with work and friends and everything. He was looking forward to running his first season of track, so we had ordered running shoes that arrived about two weeks before the schools closed.

Because they are 16 and 12, they can do a lot for themselves. They are conscientious students, and I do no homeschooling of them at all, and they seem to be keeping up with their work from school—and my 10th grader in particular has quite a lot of it—and staying occupied while my husband and I are working.

Most important, they are good company for each other. I do not mean to talk down on the experiences of only children—at one point or other, I think all of us in our house have wished we had been Onlys—but I have to say that right now, in this moment, I am particularly glad for my children that they have each other. So, my hope is that years from now, they will look back at this time and remember not just the strangeness and sadness of this moment and spending so much time on screens and missing their friends, but also that they got to be together and enjoy having a brother/sister who would walk, ride bikes, sing along to the same songs. So, maybe that will be a happy memory from now.

Quarantine quietness

April 20, 2020

GABRIELLE STOETZNER

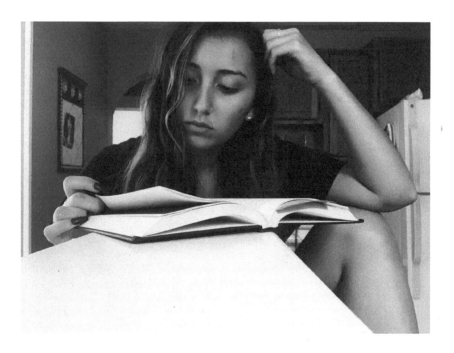

Unable to go home, I have been living on my own in Oneonta for a little over a month now. It's very different going from living in a house of four girls to being alone. It is so quiet here; I feel like I am going mad. Usually, when I'm bored, I'll just hop on my phone or laptop and scroll through social media until my eyes hurt, but that's no longer the case. Recently, logging on to social media and reading about COVID-19 has been making me feel sick to my stomach. Although it's good to stay informed about the virus, I can't help but feel scared and anxious every time I come across an update. To help me stay sane, I've tried to lay off on social media as much as I can. Instead, I try to find other things to do, such as picking up a book, cook, clean, paint and most importantly take naps.

From Afar

April 20, 2020

MATTHEW C. HENDLEY

Most of my family lives across the New York/Ontario border in Canada. I have long been accustomed to crossing the border to visit. Piling into the family van for our summer road trips to Canada is an annual tradition for us. It is about a 9- to10-hour trip from Oneonta to see my relatives in the province of Ontario (when all the rest breaks and meal breaks are added on). The border never seemed to be any major impediment. At worst, it meant a 1-hour wait to clear customs on a busy day. However, the pandemic has made the border all too real. When there is bad news from afar it is more difficult to process.

My sister who lives in Canada has been diagnosed with COVID-19. Fortunately, it seems to be a mild case. She was diagnosed through tele-medicine. Since it is not a severe case, she has not been given a COVID-19 test in accordance with policy in the province of Ontario. She is suffering from fever, aches and pains and lethargy. Thus far she has no major issues with shortness of breath or coughing. However, any COVID-19 in the family is deeply worrisome. When distance intervenes, worry increases. I have been in frequent communication with my sister and parents. I worry about how her family is coping. She is isolated in the attic room of her house. Her husband is dealing with their two active children while also trying to work from home. My parents, who are both about 80, have left some supplies on my sister's porch but can't enter the house. I feel a bit helpless being so far removed.

My family's COVID-19 situation has got me thinking about how people dealt with distant emergencies and crises in the past. My grandfather was in the US Navy in World War Two and fought in the Pacific. He left his family in Wisconsin and could only communicate with them from afar by the occasional letter. The situation of my grandparents and their children was not unique. Throughout history, many families have sent their loved ones away to war or foreign service and have waited patiently for them to come home safe. They probably only got small bits of news from their loved ones and tried not to think too much about how the global crisis might affect their family.

Our modern globalized world likes to believe that distance and borders do not matter. Technology has supposedly erased distance. Before the pandemic experts liked to say, "The world is flat"; not literally but in the sense that it was more open and accessible than ever before. You can easily be in communication with anyone anywhere at any time. Borders are irrelevant. We can travel and work in different countries. However, this pandemic is both confirming and undermining those past truisms. For COVID-19 borders and distance don't matter. It is a globalized virus. It has circled the globe and is flaring up everywhere. Within a year there will be nowhere immune from it. However, for the people stuck in the middle of the pandemic borders and distance do matter. The US/Canada border, the longest undefended border in the world, is closed. This pattern has been repeated all over the world. We are supposed to minimize unnecessary travel. Distance has re-emerged. My world has shrunk to working from home, walking around the block, and going to the grocery store once a week.

What this means is that now once again we listen to news from afar and we cannot do much more than worry. It gives me new admiration for my grandparents' generation. I think of them as I wait and hope for my sister's recovery.

Celebrating 21st birthday under quarantine

April 20, 2020

GABRIELLE BUSH

Waking up to snow in April on my birthday.

A birthday during quarantine is one of the strangest and most isolating feelings. Normally it is a day to gather with family and share a meal together. This year was very different, my parents stood at the door with masks. They visited for a few minutes and left. I never saw my grandparents or extended family and friends.

It was sad.

Definitely not how I would have imagined my 21st birthday. But in the end, it was a good day in isolation. And we restocked our quarantine supplies!

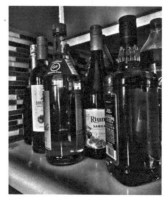

Salud!

Almost A month in . . .

April 20, 2020

CECILLE RUIZ

Today we went out. It was a good day, even if others might be mad for what I went out to do. I went to pick up my car that I bought from a sketchy man about a month ago. I bought it before this pandemic. It has less than 95,000 miles on it and it only costs about $4200. At the time I could spare that kind of money. I should have waited to make the purchase, for many reasons. Anyway, it was a good day because I got to go outside, and I got to drive! Man! I miss driving and having my music loud with the windows down and my left hand feeling the wind, the freedom. It's literally nothing, but it's one of my simplest pleasures in life. I can't wait for everything to go back to normal. I am so bored at home and so tired of seeing the same four faces every day. I go outside on a regular basis, but I miss seeing other people and being able to talk with strangers without all the panic and hysteria. Now, going outside is a hostile environment with people being ruder than ever. (Ruder sounds weird . . . I wonder if it's even a real word.) I have stress and I need the economy to get back to normal so my stress levels can go back to normal. Well, this is my good day lol.

Night.

April 20, 2020

NADIA BOYEA

Nighttime seems to be when I'm most productive since we began to quarantine. I find myself sleeping a lot during the day but am more awake at night. Time doesn't seem to go as slow when the sun isn't out. Mental health is something of concern in my household, and the hours I've been holding don't really help those concerns. I guess driving around at night is what makes me feel reminded that people are still alive; seeing lights on in all the houses is a comforting feeling even though you don't see the faces to accompany them.

What Message would this give me ten years ago?

April 20, 2020

With all the closures going on, and the kids not being in school now for over a month, I wonder what message this is giving to our children with special needs.

I'm an individual with autism. Something many of us on the spectrum face is a lack of willingness to socialize. Of the many therapies I had as a kid, one of them was designed to improve my social skills by using scenarios and having the popular kids follow me around at lunch. In elementary school, I hated it. But now, as a senior who seems to know everybody, I rely on others for my energy. I went from not wanting to leave the house, to feeling like I needed to be somewhere every day.

Last semester, I revisited some repressed thoughts I had during my period of mental crisis in middle school. There were elements of my anguish that I hadn't shaken off for years, and I finally began to find the tools to fix them. I had friends, now I needed to find meaning in my friendships. Then with the shutdowns all happening in the span of hours, everything I seemed to be working towards was rendered useless.

So that leads me to wonder what messages this is giving to the autistic kids who are still getting hold of these things. Without a doubt, some of them are probably rejoicing that they don't have to make an effort to see people. But for many of us, it's very difficult to grasp the reasoning for why things are happening in the world. For somebody to be told they have to talk to more people, only to now hear that they can't see anyone even if they wanted to, is awfully confusing. I can't be the only one who now feels their whole life is a lie, but it's definitely affecting me.

Optimism

April 20, 2020

CINDI HALL

Forever the optimist, I believe that a blessing always emerges out of something terrible. Coronavirus is horrible and scary, but I have noticed a few things during this quarantine. People are enjoying nature more, spending quality time with their loved ones, being more creative and inventive, simplifying their lives, taking naps 😴 , appreciating their health, and learning new things like how to cook, cut hair, teach, or sew. They are also stepping up to help others, checking on their neighbors, sharing resources, sending actual cards to nursing homes 👵 , and talking to God. We took so many things for granted—abundance of food, freedom to go out as we choose, and our health. My question is, why weren't we doing this all along? Maybe God or the Earth is angry, and this is our wake-up call; one last chance to change the future of our beloved planet. Perhaps we should pay attention.

An eventful quarantine day

April 21, 2020

Franklyn Macario

It wasn't a normal quarantine day. My 4 older brothers and I started the day by building a shed in the backyard for my dad. As we were working, my mom began dinner by making her famous burgers and ribs. We all gathered around the table after we were done working and enjoyed our meal as a family.

Days like today were rare before quarantine.

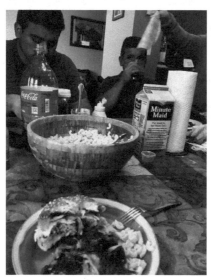

Sunday Dinner

After dinner, my best friend called me and told me he was outside. I forgot we had planned to go to a Hempstead Lake Park to walk around and see a few of our other friends. Of course, we all took the steps we needed to take in order to stay safe.

We walked around for a few hours, cracking jokes, and talking about all the plans we have after quarantine is over. We walked by this pond that seemed so peaceful and so contrary to what was happening in the world around us. I stood there for a little, trying to take it all in as much as possible. Beautiful.

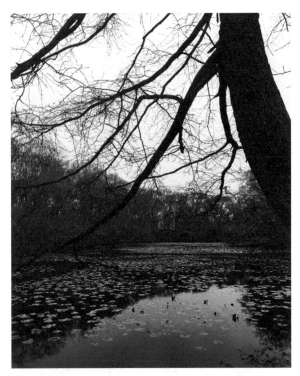

Quiet, Peaceful Pond

Thank You

April 21, 2020

ADRIANNA NEWELL

I frequently walk my dogs and go on walks around my neighborhood. Recently signs have popped up thanking essential workers and even though it is a small gesture, it is so powerful! Thank you to our essential workers!

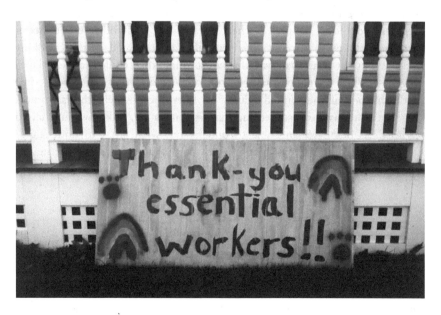

Pandemic diaries

April 22, 2020

Christina Avana

DAY 1

A Pandemic, something I have not experienced in my life before, well at least that I would be able to remember detail by detail forever. While the events on 9/11 happened when I was born, so I didn't experience it firsthand, I know that many lives were taken and effected by this. Looking back, I thought that that was the worst thing that could happen. Until now . . . While I am not making light of 9/11 and this is an awful time in the history of the United States, we knew from where this stemmed. This, the Coronavirus is something that we cannot see, unknown, uncharted territory. As being 19 and able to understand, what am I to understand? One day I am up at school getting ready for Spring break, and the next, I am quarantined in my home, with my family.

DAY 2

Nonstop news about the coronavirus. Not enough information. Where did it come from, who caused it, all speculation? The Chinese Virus it's called. Something created in China and effected the whole world. How can something affect the World? A Global pandemic. What am I to do with these words? I am not alone. Everyone is asking the same question with no answer. This is not my fault; I cannot control the outcome of this. Is this the fate of the world?

It's spreading, Italy has over 60 cases reported in a 24-hour time frame. People are dying all over. Sadness, gloom, despair, depression is setting in. If people are dying there in these great numbers, what is happening here? It's bad here, but not with those kinds of numbers. It's coming, something bad, something worse. Grandparents, parents, aunts, uncles, brothers and sisters, they're dying. Is this an apocalypse? The end of the human race? This is like watching a movie. Unreal, a sense of loneliness. I can't explain, it. People are here in my house; how can I be lonely?

Coronavirus is shutting down schools. Schools are now closed, possibly for the remainder of the semester. Online classes are to begin soon. What will that be like? It's hard to have classes with no personal interaction, at least for me. The tensions are mounting, the pressure is building, and I do not like feeling this way. Can't get my work done with all the distractions.

DAY 3

My parents are wearing masks and gloves when they go in and out the stores. Sometimes they get what they need and sometimes not. Supermarkets are working around the clock to keep shelves stocked as people are buying as if they are building a panic room or bomb shelters. There is no toilet paper, paper towels, hand sanitizer and Lysol around. The shelves are empty. Panic buying and people hoarding add stress to the trip to the grocery store. For now, my parents seem to get what they need and aside from eating take-out or making different foods, we are making do with what we have in the house and are not starving. I really believe that this will not come to pass. There is plenty of food in this world and I would really be surprised if we run out. Thank goodness for farmers.

DAY 4

My parents are in a state of disarray. Calm to the eye, but chaos inside. My family owns a transportation company, which now seems to be the forgotten industry as people are putting it. No work, no money, nothing is coming in. Quarantined in the house full of crazy people. A brother that shows no concern, a sister is more concerned overeating and tie-dying her clothing than anything, a mother that is on the phone calling no one that answers, and a father that plays games on the computer all day and sleeps the day away. Easy way to forget what's going on.

DAY 5

Social distancing, this is new. You have to keep space between yourself and other people. They recommend staying at least 6 feet from other people, do not gather in groups, stay out of crowded places.

What happened to my friends? I haven't really seen anyone in a while. I went to the beach and met up with some friends. We sat in our separate cars and talked through the windows. 6 feet apart in separate cars is really hard to do. You never think about this until you actually have to do it. We drink coffee and discussed, what? Nothing. All of a sudden, we have nothing to discuss besides this virus. Things are unimportant these days. Words are meaningless and pointless, there is nothing to look forward to until this pandemic comes to an end. When will that be, there is no date in sight?

Don't even know what day it is. Days are going into one another. Information on the internet or on the news is more detailed these days. Or maybe not. Contradictory conversations are all over the place. No one seems to be on the same page. The President says that everything is good and beautiful, while the doctors are making a little headway in a cure. Information is misguided. My parents' concerns are growing stronger.

Shelter in place. Stay wherever you are, at home, until the threat is over during the COVID-19 pandemic to help prevent the spread of disease. This can be months. The thought of this lasting months is a nail biter!

DAY 6

We decided as a family that we would not watch the news on the television all day. We've talked about the virus and how we have to stay home and be safe. I overheard some conversations between my mom and dad talking about people being hospitalized, death tolls and fears for our friends and family. We have family affected by this and I am sad, scared, and helpless. I can only help at this point by sending our thoughts and prayers to those affected by this disease and let my family know that I am here for them and thinking about them.

Anxiety, maybe not for some, although I don't understand how not everyone, but for others, the psychological stress, the constant worry, crazy unpleasant thoughts that run through your mind, boredom. Trying not to think of it. I do my homework and my assignments, and I go move on. Watching my 2-year-old cousin is a distraction, so that helps. But then he goes home and here I am . . . bed to couch to kitchen table to bed. Too much time to reflect on what I am feeling about all these uncertainties.

OMG tomorrow is another day.

DAY 7

How to get through a quiet day? Binge watch episodes of the Kardashians and Vampire Diaries. I saw them all already, nothing like repetition, no cliffhangers here, but it helps with the not sleeping, tiredness, and continuous eating, what could be worse? Is this my new addiction? I thought it was chickpeas!!

I miss school and I miss my friends. Being stuck at home for this long is torture. Having contact with my family only causes nothing but fights, it's horrible. I miss my old life. College was my safe place. I cannot wait to be let out of this lockdown. The second it's over is the second I leave for days and never stay in this house again, it's bad. All I do is fight with my siblings. My brothers are annoying and rude, my dad's loud and my sister is just an annoyance. No one understands the fact that I'm not on break, I have homework and class work and I AM STILL IN SCHOOL. This isn't my free time, I can never get anything done without my dad speaking, it's extremely annoying. I need out of this house before I go absolutely insane.

DAY 8

Taking a deep breath. Heard on the news this morning that the number of confirmed people leaving the hospital is getting higher. That's a good thing. Did we reach a peak? People are getting better and that makes me happy to hear positive news instead of only concentrating on negative reports.

So, my nails are a disaster. What to do? All the nail salons are closed. Idea, have my mother give me a manicure. Hey exciting, something different to do. Okay, not the best decision I've made so far, polish all over my skin, bumps in the polish, nails filed crooked and changed the color several times. For what, no one can see it anyway, oh well, just because.

Ok so I wanted a drink, I went to the cabinet to get a cup and took out a paper plate. What was I thinking, oh yeah, I'm not!! I'm going crazy.

DAY 9

I need out of this house, it's getting worse. No one stops fighting!! Too much family time going on. We all need to go our separate ways but there's nowhere to go!! What am I going to do? I need to see my friends and I need to go outside and relax. I need to drive around with my friends and blast music on the parkway to the beach. I need to go out and party with my friends or just meet up with everyone and have a chill day. This whole facetime thing every night is not doing it for me. I am dying of boredom. I NEED OUT!!!!

DAY 10

I miss my old life, before this virus. I miss my freedom. I miss Oneonta and doing what I want when I want to. I miss seeing my friends every day and going out with them or watching movies. I miss not being told what to do or being annoyed by my siblings. I miss my independence and I cannot wait for this to be over to get that back for the remainder of the time I'm home and so on in college. Sophomore year is approaching as freshman year starts coming to an end. We don't even know what our rooming situation is yet because were all sidetracked and behind. This is insane, I hope things get better within this month. It needs to.

Easter time amid a pandemic

April 22, 2020

JOSEPH SUHOVSKY

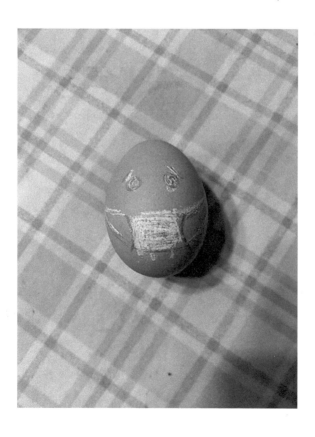

Grocery Store Diaries

April 22, 2020

COURTNEY JONES

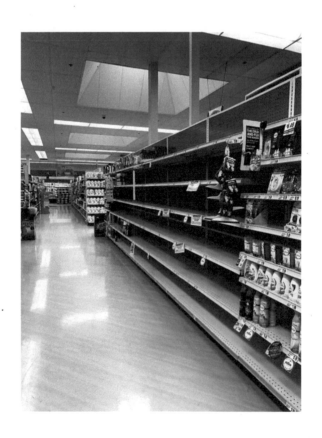

Best time to have a pet

April 22, 2020

MARIA CRISTINA MONTOYA

I never had a pet before in my life; my first dog came last year during a challenging time in my life and ironically, he came at the right moment to continue helping my family in challenging times. He is the center of our home now, he takes us out of the house to play, hike and walk. All will be better soon.

The joy in these times

April 22, 2020

MICHAEL ACQUAFREDDA

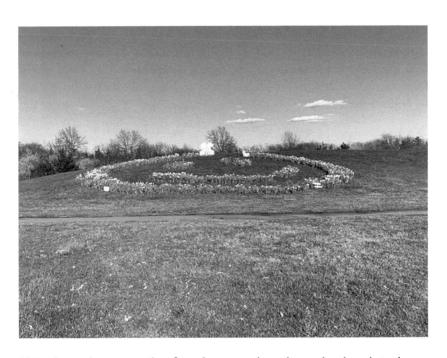

This photo shows a smiley face that was planted at a local park in hopes to cheer people up during this time of distress.

Small Things

April 22, 2020

KIM SE-CHAN

Being intensely quarantined for 14 days has taught me things. Things that are not always apparent in normal life. It's the details that matter.

If you look at any object closely, not even little parts are made by mistake. They all have purpose and function.

When we apply this idea on a larger scale, we can rethink the meaning of society. We all see society as a huge machine, but looking at the current situation, it is individual people who actually run the machine.

This principle is true for every phenomenon. If we want to achieve something big, we need everyone's support. Everyone counts.

I am starting to get sick of the word, Corona, or COVID-19. Let's do our part and get over this phase.

Introduction . . .

April 23, 2020

Cecille Ruiz

Hey! This is my second entry, probably a little late for intros, but better late than never! My name is Cecille Ruiz. I am from Hudson, NY (the cutest little city in Eastern New York). Well, I guess I will tell you a little about myself, so you can understand my point of view. My favorite colors are blue and pink just like cotton candy. I worked two jobs on campus, back when we were still on campus. I miss my jobs, sometimes. I prefer working in real life as opposed to this whole virtual reality life I feel like I'm in. I hope things go back to normal soon. I went for a walk the other day with my family to get some food. This lady was also walking up the street and she said, "I think you all should be walking in a single file line." There's four of us, by the way. We were so shocked we all stood there staring at her confused. LOL. We were in such shock we didn't know what to say. We all stood there staring back at each other, I think she was waiting for us to move first. LOL. I laugh every time I think back to this. We just left because we didn't know what to say, but then later we thought of a bunch of funny things. That was off topic, but I don't really know what to say. I have so much I want to say, but I have no idea where to start. Oh, by the way, I am Mexican, 20 years old (I turn 21 in JUNE!), I do have white skin, though, so don't picture any stereotypes. I have two loving parents, and two younger siblings and my major is Psychology. I can't wait for summer! I love the warmth of the sun on my face. Okay, well, that's all I can think of. I will keep you updated when I think of more things to say. Ciao!

Last week

April 23, 2020

Nadia Boyea

This past week I was out in my car and outside for a walk. Cars still passed by somewhat frequently, but there were certainly not as many people out in the towns I drove through. It snowed overnight one night and that felt very fitting for the mood, even though it's April. The day before the snow, it felt bitter and dreary and gloomy out, like you knew the snow was coming. Unlike the snow, we didn't know that all of this was about to happen to us. All we can do is take it day by day and hope for the best outcome.

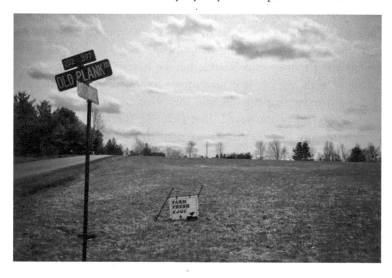

What day is it?

April 23, 2020

KELLY N. TENBUS

I feel like days keep on passing by. I try to do stuff like work out or read a book and keep up with my schoolwork, but nothing interesting is happening. I call my friends and we just talk about how online school sucks, the things we do to attempt to stay busy, and the boredom we face every single day. I feel like the day happens and I am not present for it. I'm not dissociating or anything, but nothing feels productive or rewarding. A day starts and ends, but nothing has changed. The only thing that does change is the news gets worse. President Trump keeps lying to himself and the country saying it will be over soon. Last month he said it would be done by Easter, I don't think many people believed him. Recently, he stopped putting money into WHO, but he never listened to scientists if they disagree with him, so it is no surprise (example: the mess he made of EPA). I heard today that the UK said they would have social distancing in place until the end of the year!!! That feels like forever away. But there is no vaccine or cure for COVID-19 so until those arrive there really is no guarantee any of this will end soon. I think by the end of this the entire world will be depressed.

Another Thursday . . .

April 25, 2020

CECILLE RUIZ

Hey readers! LOL. I like imagining I have a ton of fans out there reading my posts. I'm posting kind of late at night, but I spent all day doing schoolwork. I was talking to a friend yesterday and she said something I thought was very relatable. She said, "It feels like there's more work now, than there was when we were at school." I absolutely agree! I feel like I had so much more free time back in Oney! I was super stressed today, though, not only from schoolwork, but also from real life problems. I gotta figure out what I'm gonna do for summer work. Bills keep coming and no one gives 2 f***s about people struggling financially in this epidemic. I don't really curse a lot, I cringe when I do, but I get so mad/frustrated sometimes and it slips out. This may be a long entry, but I just gotta vent. Anyway, back to bills and financial stress. My mom got laid off also because of this epidemic. My dad's the only one working right now. I'm concerned because she's been dipping into her savings for rent. Sometimes I wanna cry out of frustration for how helpless I feel. I know crying is not weakness, and I respect those who can show their emotions in front of people, that's bravery. Unfortunately, crying doesn't fix anything, though, so if I were to cry, I would just feel useless and I probably wouldn't be able to stop, honestly. Haha, probably TMI, oh well! I didn't get to work out today, I think that may be why I have so much negative vibes. I haven't smoked in over two months and times like these I could really use a smoke on the roof. It's something me and my housemates used to do back in Oney. I can't smoke when I'm home: Life's a struggle, but oh well. Anyway, I've also been really stressed because I'm gonna be a senior next year and I AM NOT READY TO GROW UP. I used to have a plan. My plan was I would graduate high school, go to college, major in psych, graduate college with some kind of honors, go straight into the Peace Corps about a month or two after, then go to grad school and then figure out what to do with my life. It's crazy that life really doesn't go the way you plan, no matter how hard you try staying on track. I don't want to join the Peace Corps anymore. I would like to help people, but I'm afraid of growing up, honestly. Well, I'll write another entry on my future life plans after this, for now I will vent. I have come to the conclusion that me and my brother will have to get jobs ASAP and my mother can stay and watch my sister. I am also very stressed because I had bought a car from a random person before this s**t happened and now I can't even drive it around because I was never able to register it and switch the license plates and change the title. I'm stressed because I keep getting this thought in the back of my head, 'what if I bought a stolen car?? and the guy just ran off with the money???' I'm a little nervous because even though this sounds cocky, I am never wrong, even when I wish I was. I have a sixth sense of knowing everything, and it's a blessing and a curse. Okay, I'm gonna move on, I hate talking about my problems. It's pointless if no one's gonna solve them for me. Side note: I am not a negative Nancy, I'm only negative in my mind and I'm typing literally as I think. Also, I had some revelations I'll share in my next entry, this one's already super long.

Indoors

April 27, 2020

MARIA CRISTINA MONTOYA

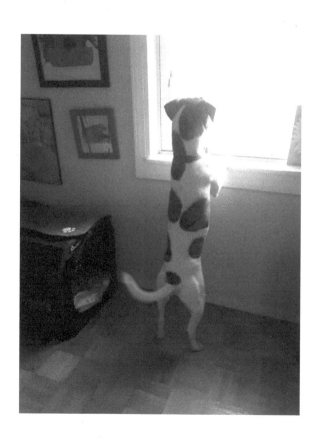

Descending or Ascending?

April 27, 2020

WESLEY BERNARD

This has been a week of deep despair and tragedy for some of my students. And yet at the same time, some have shown resiliency, tenacity, and hope in spite of it all.

It makes me wonder which way we are headed as a nation. I think Ascending.

Home life

April 27, 2020

MOLLY JEAN FEULNER

Hello everyone, my name is Molly Feulner. I'm fairly new to the Oneonta family, I returned to school last fall after an absence of five years to finish my degree in Fine Arts. My focus is photography, so I wanted to share with you my documentation of this time. This series of self-portraits shows how I have been spending my time in isolation. I have started a larger project I will share when I have completed it.

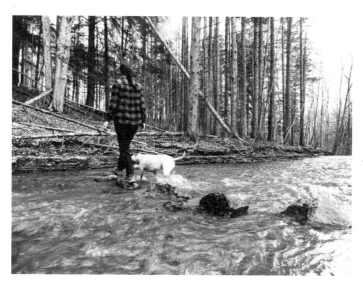

Spending lots of time grooming hiking/biking trails in the woods near my house. My dogs are enjoying us being home so much and the frequent walks in the woods. My fiancé made these steps for us to cross the creek and work on our trails through the woods.

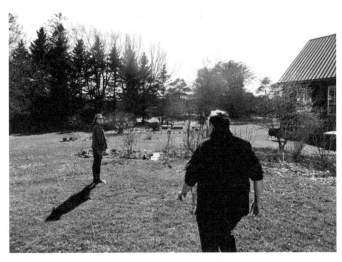

Visiting my parents' home, meeting them outside, practicing social distancing.

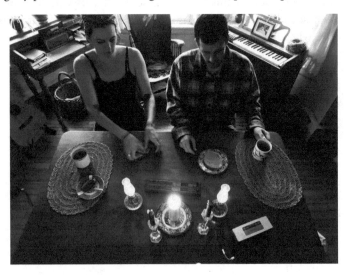

Lots of time has been spent playing card and dice games in the dining room. I am planning my wedding for this summer. I love origami and decided to make all of the invitations by hand using origami designs.

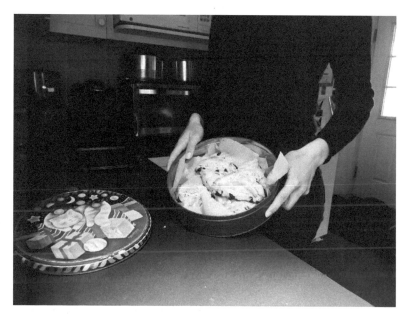

I love to bake as well, lots of scones and cookies being consumed around here! I've experienced lots of ups and downs through this time. On the one hand, I do have introvert tendencies, so spending lots of time at home doesn't bother me very much. I find it easy to fill my time with hobbies that I enjoy and normally don't have that much time for. On the other hand, not being able to spend time with friends in my home or theirs, going to the grocery store and the gas station have become incredibly stressful things for me. I have had pneumonia a number of times in my short life and truly fear contracting this disease and becoming gravely ill. It's a strange feeling being pulled in both directions, longing for my friends and family's company while also fearing being around anyone.

Last Week

April 27, 2020

KIM SE-CHAN

It has been confusing for a few weeks, and I am thankful that nothing serious happened to me. The coming week is going to be my last week in the US. After that, I am leaving for Korea. Fortunately, Korea's situation is getting better, but I'm not totally comfortable leaving the US in this circumstance. Even though the light at the end of the tunnel seems to fade away, I will keep praying for Oneonta and the US for stableness. I hope the continuing losses will soon cease and recover from this depression. Later, I believe, there will be a time we will remember this with loved ones and keep living as we did before the virus.

End of the semester worries

April 28, 2020

Gabrielle Bush

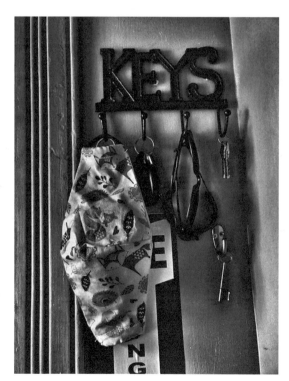

Keep my mask by my keys

As the semester comes to an end, I am grateful to soon be finished with online classes. However, uncertainty makes me fearful. Quarantine had been difficult even with keeping busy with schoolwork, but now that is ending, and I still do not have a job. I fear for the days to come until places open up and I can get one. What will I do? How will I keep myself busy and out of bed?

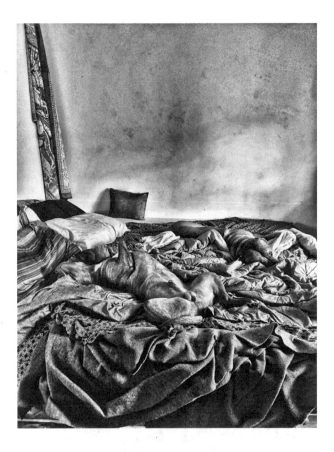

I worry about getting a job during these times. Having a compromised immune system and struggling every day with my health, what job could I possibly hold?

Times of uncertainty are difficult to face. As of now, I look forward to life being back to normal soon and enjoy getting outside as much as I can.

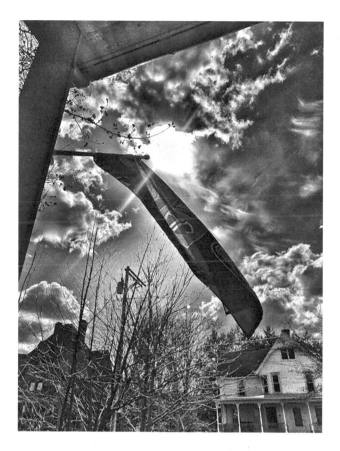

Until then, this is our new normal.

20 Years in 2 weeks

April 28, 2020

JIM GREENBERG

The last twenty years of my career at the College were spent, in part, participating in putting in place the resources to teach online. Not always an easy or valued thing. SUNY Oneonta, with good reason, prides itself on being a quality, *traditional*, teaching institution. Teaching online was mostly viewed with skepticism.

You can imagine then that after **twenty years** I watched (from the safety of retirement) with sympathy as everyone went to online learning in just **two weeks**. Not just the students and faculty, but support systems like the library, student tutoring, registration, student advisement, etc. Stunning really and as some would say, tragically ironic. It is almost by chance that the pieces for online learning were left intact allowing the campus to continue to offer courses during the pandemic. It is also a testament to the entire campus community they were able to pull this off.

My office during quarantine, Suite 203,
South Side Hall, SUNY Oneonta.

April 28, 2020

Maria Cristina Montoya

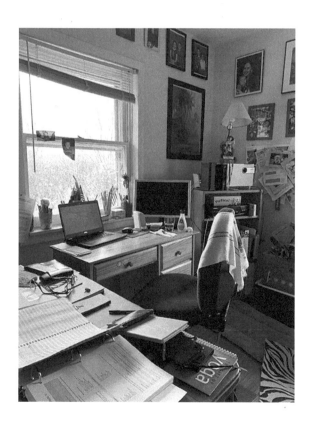

A new perspective

April 29, 2020

GABRIELLE STOETZNER

Last week, I posted an update to this blog called "Quarantine Quietness." I talked about how I had been going crazy trying to keep myself occupied while living in Oneonta alone. Since then, one of my housemates decided to move back in and quarantine with me. Upon her arrival, I noticed a dramatic change in my mental state, and I now have someone to be crazy with. From dying hair crazy colors to playing guitar hero until 2 am, I am so grateful to have her back.

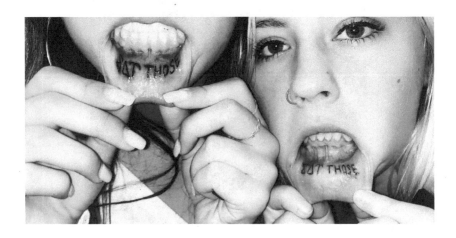

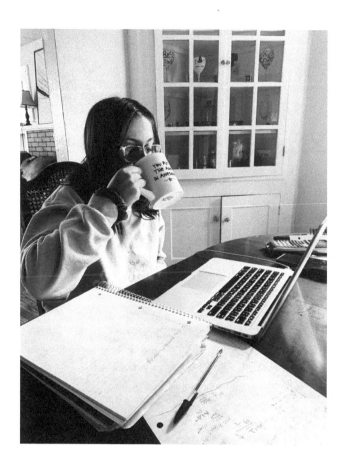

Hope

April 29, 2020

James R. Ebert

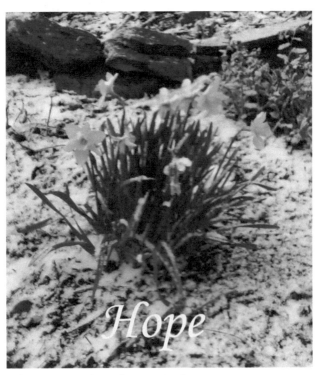

A message from our garden after an April snow.

Life at home

April 30, 2020

SAMANTHA ARNOLD

The quarantine has been especially hard for me and my family. It started out with not being able to go to the store, then it turned into not being able to go anywhere, not even to my fiancé's house. After about a week of being in quarantine, my grandma gave us the news that her cancer had come back. She had full intentions of getting chemotherapy and attending my wedding in the summer of 2021. She wanted to fight her cancer until she landed in the hospital because of her cancer. While there, she could not have any visitors and she, along with the nurses and doctors, had to wear a mask. She was so scared and wanted to come home. After running a few tests, they let her come home and two days after that, she went to her chemotherapy appointment. She was scared to go, scared to go through chemotherapy for the second time within less than five years. She asked the doctor some questions while there and realized she could not go through it again. The side effects were too scary, potentially enough to kill her after just one dose. She decided, being 81, that she would rather spend her last days with her family. It has been three weeks now that she has been in Hospice at home. My family and I have been helping her all day and every day. She is so grateful for us and she is so happy she lived a full life with love and happiness. I know the end is coming for her and I am so scared. I wanted her to be at my wedding and I did not see this coming. I tried on her wedding dress, along with my mother's and my aunt's, just so she could feel like she was a part of it all. She told me although she won't be there in person, she will still be there. I hope that is the truth, I hope I will be able to feel her presence. I can't wait for this virus to be over, for me to finish grieving over my grandma, and for things to get back to normal. I pray for that day.

3

May 2020

SUNY ONEONTA

May 6—Last day of spring 2020 final exam period. The semester is finally over!

ONEONTA

May 20—Otsego County marks three weeks with no COVID cases.

May 20—Otsego County Board of Representatives votes to lay off fifty-nine county employees to cut costs and save money due to massive budget impact of COVID.

May 29—Second phase of reopening authorized for "nonessential" Otsego County businesses due to declining rates of COVID.

May 31—Hundreds rally in Muller Plaza in Oneonta to protest death of George Floyd.

NEW YORK

May 14—Statewide State of Emergency extended to June 13.

May 23—Gatherings of up to ten people are now allowed as long as social distancing is practiced.

USA

May 22—The United States remains the global epicenter with more than 1.6 million cases and the number of deaths nearing 100,000.

May 25—Murder of George Floyd by Minneapolis police officer Derek Chauvin.

May 27—Deaths from COVID-19 surpass the 100,000 mark.

WORLD

May 17—Japan and Germany, two of the world's largest economies, enter recessions.

Wild Life

May 1, 2020

Matthew C. Hendley

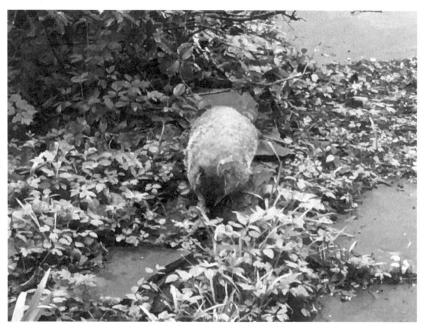

The Groundhog in action

WILD LIFE

There are certain moments when you realize that everything you always assumed about the natural world was wrong. I knew that the pandemic had really changed things when I saw a massive furry beast in my backyard. A few mornings ago, I opened our downstairs blind and saw a groundhog the size of a small dog calmly staring back at me less than ten feet away. In the bright sunlight it was having a nice breakfast by eating our grass and back garden. Though the sight of this intruder was unusual, its attitude was what was most striking. It barely blinked but instead eyed me with a calm, even superior gaze. Our small fenced-in backyard has always hosted cats, squirrels, and birds. However, since we live in the heart of the city of Oneonta and are less than 3 minutes' walk from Main Street, the call of nature is usually muted for us. On ordinary mornings as we rush about to get ready for work, any groundhogs are hidden. They prefer to wait for nighttime to forage. Animals consciously avoid my family's frenetic morning routine as we heave our bags and backpacks into the van to speed to work and take our daughter to school. However, now wildlife has taken over.

When I look for items online to update myself on news about the pandemic, I often come across similar out of kilter animal images on my computer screen: Mountain goats quietly strolling through empty village streets; bears checking out dogs with nary a human to intervene; lions having a nice mid-day nap on paved roads in Africa. What does it mean? The animal kingdom, previously cowed by a loud and visible human presence, has been emboldened. As humans scurry into cover and hide indoors, the outdoors has changed.

When I was young, there was a powerful animated film I saw called *Watership Down*. As memory serves, it was about rabbits endangered by the encroachments of human development. Cars were lethal weapons to the rabbits. Bulldozers threatened their burrows. Man was out to conquer nature. Wildlife would be tamed. The animals' arcadia was to be destroyed. Many precious rabbits died. I cried childhood tears as I watched the film. This theme has been repeated in many other stories and films, but it seems to be on hold for the moment. The pandemic has shown that humans are not always all powerful. It has shown that nature can reconfigure the lives of humans and beasts.

There is one final thing that my moment with the groundhog taught me. We have always assumed that we had the freedom to go anywhere. We had machines and large brains. Animals had to adapt to us. We watched them and they hid from us. The pandemic has flipped the script. Now we hide and they watch us. Perhaps the wild ones were the wise ones all along.

Quarantine-Time

May 1, 2020

GAVIN BROWN

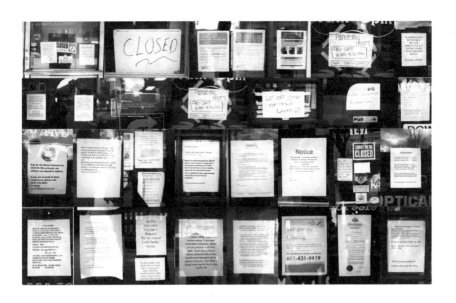

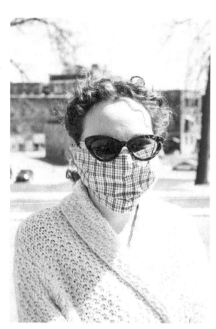
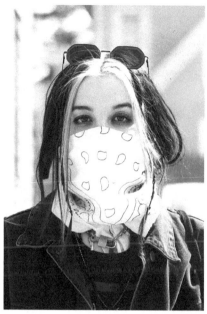
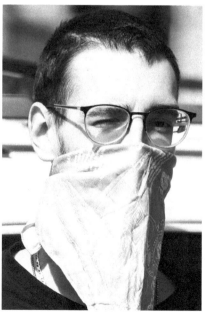
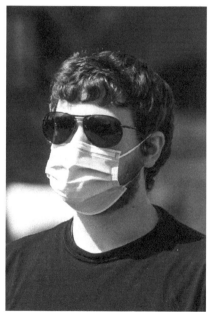

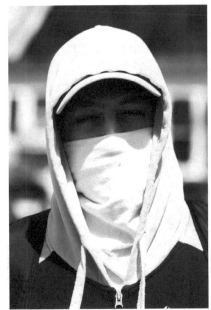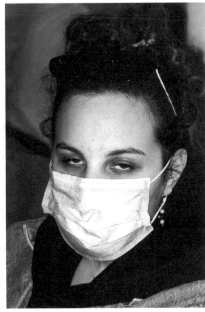

A collection of quarantine-time people, places, and activities.

Surreal but very real

May 2, 2020

HALES PINK

In the rush to get back to normal, use this time to decide which parts of normal are worth rushing back to.

—Dave Hollis

The only word I have to describe our current situation is surreal. I recall talking about the coronavirus in my classes before spring break. We thought nothing of it. Then we all leave for a break and enter our own little worlds away from college. I myself was 12 hours away from Oneonta, not thinking about responsibilities, family, or school and certainly not a virus. I was totally present in enjoying my spring vacation at the beach and playing ultimate. But on the last day of the tournament, we start sticking our heads into the real world and find out that COVID-19 is serious, and the college might be shutting down. My teammates and I were trying to wrap our heads around what was happening. We were so separated from what was going on that it felt like we were in a simulation. While we lived out the last few days of freedom, we weren't thinking that the world would be like it is right now. We were just trying to enjoy the warm weather and time with our friends to do whatever.

The next few days felt like a movie. Coming out of the best week of the year to having an extended break was like Christmas came early. But the joy didn't last long before panic and fear set in. Everyone was trying to figure out where they were staying for the rest of the semester. There were so many questions that didn't have answers. After driving 12 hours back to Oneonta, I was picked up by my parents the very next day and brought home. We packed up my dorm and said goodbye in less than an hour. One could've said we were on the run, and it would be moments before we were found. You didn't know that this would be the last time you saw someone for a while, you didn't know that this would be the last of many lasts for a while or forever.

The next couple of weeks were disorienting and confusing. All you wanted to do was go out and about, or work, or see your friends, and the world is telling you no, you're not allowed. Being someone who was having social interaction 20/7 to only seeing my family for the next who knows how long, was taking a toll on my mental, emotional, and physical health. It's frustrating and you want to blame someone but who is there to blame? The measures that have been taken are said to be unnecessary but are they really? These are lives we are talking about! It's difficult to understand but 6 feet apart is for protection. Sure, you may not think you have it, but how would you know? What if you do have it, you can easily infect every single person you come in contact with and every person who comes in contact with something you touched? The reality of this disease is so abstract and abnormal that people don't want to believe it but it's real. Very, very real.

I don't think a lot of people, especially in the beginning, entered reality. For many, this was something that would pass in a month, this was something that wasn't affected them directly so it didn't truly exist. But just because we are not face to face with COVID-19, it is very much a serious situation. People are still stuck in coming to terms with how their lives have changed and how all the measures that have been taken are for the good of the people. Until people stop focusing on the individual and start thinking about surviving this together, our world will remain in this state.

It is okay to have all the feelings. Frustration, sadness, depression, anxiety, fear. But also have happiness, love, excitement, pride, enjoyment. Accepting that this is how the world is at the moment and everyone is doing their best or should be doing their best during these times is so important. We can't let ourselves get sucked into our negative emotions. Feel them, sit in them, but don't let them consume you. Life has already been turned upside down, but you're still alive, you've still got your future, so live your days for the ones you will have when this is over. Plan like you would if we weren't living in a pandemic and know that you may have to adjust those plans, but at least if you're given the green light, you get to do what you were looking forward to doing.

Once the light turns green, it's so important to remember what it felt like to have your life turned upside down so quickly. We should focus on the problems that are actually serious. We should be grateful for the ones who stayed by our side through this all and be thankful for everything that we have. Yeah, we want to get back to our old lives, but the world is changed permanently and it's important to de-clutter ourselves so that we're focusing on the parts that are worth the time, energy, and resources that we put in.

The end

May 2, 2020

KIM SE-CHAN

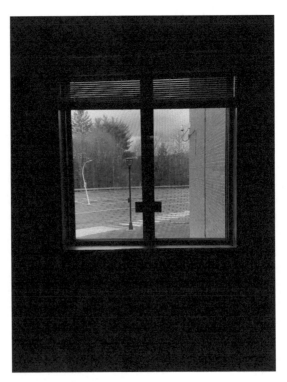

Final over . . . waiting my time to go!

Gas stations

May 3, 2020

NADIA BOYEA

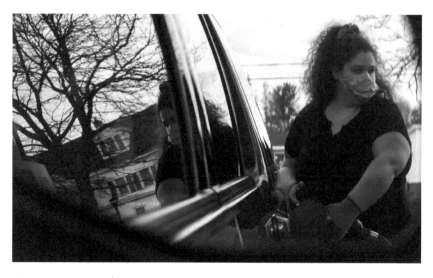

There are still a fair amount of people who are not following social distancing, nor the new law about mask requirements. Gas stations are where I see the most variation in rule followers. Tonight, I saw someone walk up to the door at Stewart's, see the sign that said a mask was required to enter and proceeded to turn around and return to their car. I still don't think people believe that all of this is helping anything, and with that mentality, they're part of why there is not better progress being made.

Measuring a month

May 3, 2020

Tyra A. Olstad

Wake, walk, eat, work; work, walk, eat, sleep. Wake in the middle of the night, work, sleep. Wake, walk.

Days and weeks have blurred together. If I didn't keep a calendar filled with reminders for "dept mtg," "sr sem presentations," "J b-day," I wouldn't know, is it Monday or Friday, already May or still mid-March? (Doesn't help that the sky continues to spit sleet.) And if I didn't also fill the calendar with memories of "rainbow," "first forsythia," "forget-me-nots," I wouldn't know, has time actually passed, anything happened other than the odd progression of the semester, the escalating panic of the news, the accumulating silence?

I'm perfectly accustomed to spending long stretches of time on my own, but voluntarily, on backpacking trips through far-flung, wild corners of the country. Disorienting, now, to be stuck pacing the same sidewalks and streets, surrounded by people, all shuttered in their homes or sealed in their cars. On rare sunny days, it's reassuring to see others out jogging in the parks or biking down the trails. But when it's raining (or sleeting), I walk through a ghost city, sidewalks to myself.

There's still the wildlife. Most of my calendar notes consist of weather or wildlife-spottings. Killdeer by Corning (4/16), beaver by the golf course (4/25), barred owl in Wilber Park (4/17), common mergansers in Neahwa (4/24). Bald eagle by the West End wetland, eagle along the river, eagle in the cemetery; eagle over the Price Chopper parking lot, infiltrating a kettle of vultures (4/29). Woodchucks everywhere—a grand one-day tally of six. Stopped counting the ravens and crows scavenging deer and squirrels from the roadsides. Dead porcupine after dead porcupine after dead porcupine, 4/7, 4/10, 4/28. (With less traffic, how is there still so much roadkill? As if there isn't enough sorrow in the world right now.)

The eagles, in particular, bring a feeling of fierce joy, a welcome reminder of perseverance and recovery. There's one that likes to perch above the railroad tracks, out River Street Access Road, next to the highway. I visit it nearly every afternoon; it lets me stand and watch it, while red-winged blackbirds swoop at it in distress and cars continue to whiz down the highway. After 5 or 10 minutes, I usually get tired, or it gets bored; we go on with our lives. Fly away. Walk, work, eat, sleep.

If the forsythia and forget-me-nots aren't enough of a clue, the calendar tells me we're nearing the end of the semester. The best advice I have, at a time like this; *especially* at a time like this; always? Even if it's sleeting, go for a walk. Watch for eagles. Brake for porcupines.

Let's all become armchair medical anthropologists

May 6, 2020

SALLIE HAN

As a medical anthropologist, I think about sickness (or health) as significantly a social and cultural experience. My perception at this moment is that while we are rightly concerned with addressing the virus (SARS-CoV-2) and the disease it causes (COVID-19), we have almost no control over the virus or over the course of the disease. Meanwhile, we are overlooking what we can do. **We have the power to change our own behaviors**, and I wish we as a public might turn our attention now to directing our efforts to reinventing our habits (and the conditions that enable or disable them) with the same urgency. That is the other part of what we need to do in order to "resume" lives that bear some resemblance to what we considered normal and ordinary before.

So many people have become armchair epidemiologists. I invite us to become medical anthropologists now 😊 .

First, let's start by valuing what we actively already have done: Those of us who have the privilege of doing so have made extraordinary changes by living in "lockdown" and "shelter in place" and adapting our activities to enable work and school from home. However, I think we all recognize this is only a temporary "stop" or "pause"—and at some point, later I want to dwell on the language and metaphors of this moment.

Next, let's recognize that culture and social change are as important and necessary to live through and beyond this moment as a vaccine against the virus and medical therapies for the disease. I've been thinking the responses around the AIDS pandemic might provide models for what needs to happen next. Obviously, HIV and SARS-CoV-2 are quite different—and in fact, SARS-CoV-2 is much more contagious! Consider, however, that we have no vaccine for HIV, but we have widespread availability of (free) testing; safe and efficacious therapies that enable HIV+ individuals to live otherwise healthy; and most importantly, changes in cultural attitudes and norms and social behaviors that prevent or at least minimize the risk of infection. These required a lot of activism and campaigning, but they happened. We have not eradicated HIV/AIDS, and infection is still a threat, but we have made considerable strides to contain it, and it is not the plague and death sentence it once was.

A quick note for now: Changing our habits is likely as hard (or even harder) than controlling the virus—I'm not suggesting culture change is easier than virology because I think there's a lot of evidence that people themselves are as stubborn as their sicknesses—but at least it's in our power to do it.

Quarantined; from the outside looking in

May 10, 2020

MOLLY JEAN FEULNER

I wanted a way to connect with my friends and family while staying safe and keeping our distance, so I decided to photograph them from the outside looking in. I also wanted to give people a space to express how they are feeling about this pandemic and being quarantined, so I asked everyone a few short questions to answer as they felt fit.

1. What are you feeling during this time? How is this affecting you personally?

2. How has this pandemic affected your job and/or schooling?

3. If you haven't been working, what have you been filling your time with? Are you able to do things you normally don't have time for?

I wanted to know how this was affecting everyone personally, their jobs, schooling, what people are doing with their time. I tried to get a range of situations, from people still working, those who were laid off, business owners, kids working on school from home, teachers, and musicians to see the range of effects on our community. Some people were more responsive than others, but I found some are being affected much more than others.

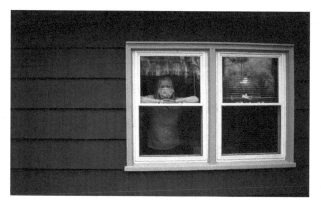

Suzanne Schnettler

PALATINE BRIDGE, NY

S: "Not much has changed for me during this pandemic. I'm fortunate enough to be able to work from home. I do miss the socialization with my co-workers though, so at times I do feel lonely working from home."

S: "I'm not getting any extra projects done at home since I spend most of the day working. I have been making masks in my spare time to hand out to people."

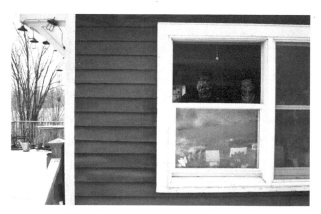

Nick Jordan + Marissa Breault

CHERRY VALLEY, NY

N: "I guess I would say that I am having lots of mixed feelings about what's going on right now. I mean, generally speaking, I sit painfully in the middle on lots of issues."

N: "I'm back in college for wildlife and fishery techniques right now. This is a very hands-on course of study, so 'distance learning' is a struggle. My other half is working from home, so we have each other and our dogs, so there is a silver lining."

N: "We've been fishing and doing lots of outdoor activities when the weather will allow, I plan on hunting turkeys no different than I ever would. There are lots of perks to living in the country, being away from lots of people and the type of panic that can bring is just the tip of the iceberg."

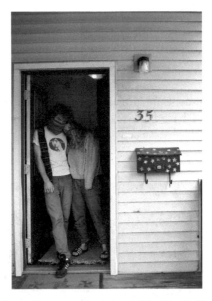

Jack Loewenguth + Mikala Gallo

ONEONTA, NY

M: "This time has surfaced many different feelings for both of us. I think from the beginning of this all, I'd say late February to now, we've experienced drastic change in our ideologies on how to approach the current situation. It has been a constant shift over months of confusion and sometimes chaos.

However, this pause has been a welcomed break in many ways; the time and space to reflect as well as relax at moments has also been soothing and helpful. That's not to say we don't feel the intense frustration and unease this all has created for our community. We also feel thankful and fortunate that we can stay home with our pup."

M: "This pandemic has forced both of us to stay home. Jack works at a gym which has been mandated to be closed until further notice, without pay. I (Mikala) have been home since March 17th, and I am still receiving pay. I'm supposed to return to work May 15th, though it has been pushed back at least 3 times. We both agree that one of the most challenging pieces to this all is the unknown of when things will shift into a more socially 'open' phase."

M: "We've been spending a lot of time cooking, watching shows/movies, hiking, playing Super Smash Bro's, creating art, and crying. It's been a stew of everything really."

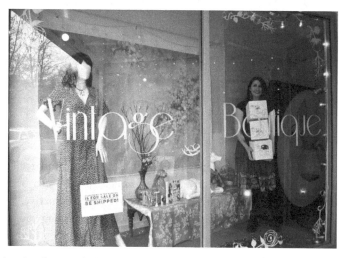

Elizabeth Raphelson (Owner of The Underground Attic)

ONEONTA, NY

E: "I am feeling quite literally everything during this time. Roller coaster doesn't begin to describe it. I feel thankful for my privilege, I feel sorry for the loss of so many people, I miss some of the things I do regularly that make me happy; I feel determined to make this time special."

E: "This pandemic has meant my brick-and-mortar shop is closed. Same with my boyfriend who has a shop right next door. This is of course very scary, but I'm trying to do as much as I can with online sales and hope that I come out the other side having improved my business."

E: "I am working, but during free time I have been reading, exercising and doing creative activities like dancing and music!"

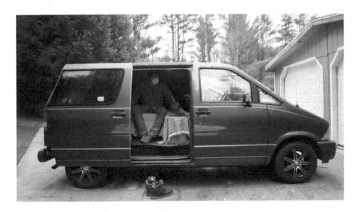

Evan Jagels

Hartwick, NY

E: "I've been missing the varieties of human interaction and realizing the importance of a positive perspective. For example, isolation can be negative and daunting, while solitude can be contemplative and productive. Knowing that the whole world is in this together has been comforting too."

E: "Innovation comes out of necessity and as an educator, this has forced me to adopt new methods of instruction and assessment. Some of these I will take with me when we return to the classroom. However, over half of my income comes from performing. Separate from the income, making music for and with people has such immensely positive social and emotional benefits that I am deeply missing. It's largely who I am, and that has been suspended indefinitely."

E: "My biggest hobby is things that move. Luckily, I was able to order a lot of parts during the onset of everything and I have gotten a lot of work done on my motorcycles and my van. I am a bit of a gym rat, swimmer, and rock climber and have been finding new ways to stay active and exercise using what I have on my property. I've also been spending more time doing visual art, and, of course, practicing music and collaborating with friends and colleagues all over the world on some fun and interesting music projects."

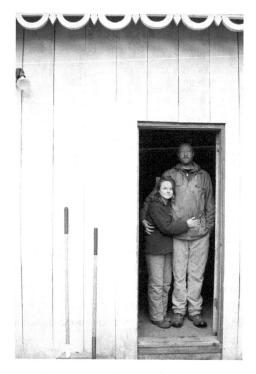

Lorry O'Brien Dubois + Jackson Dubois

WESTVILLE, NY

J: "I feel incredibly grateful to be hunkered down at a high point in my life, it could have happened at any time. I feel sadness for what the world is going through and that feels emotionally raw at times."

J: "I am working from home. It's been a bit of a challenge, many of my coworkers are laid off and that feels like a big responsibility."

J: "I imagined having lots of time to work in the garden or on my house, but it really requires fairly strict time management to get anything done. I see the amount of work that this old place would have required as a farm without engines and primitive machinery."

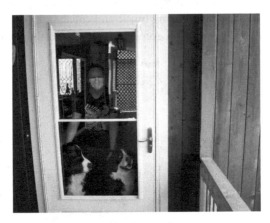

Josh Cornish

Milford, NY

J: "I feel that isolation has been difficult because I like to socialize at SUCO with classmates and professors. I think the thing I miss most of all is hanging with friends although I have had a lot of board game nights recently, which have helped during the quarantine. I feel as though this has shown me that I could not take online classes and could not have done it without my professors."

J: "Seem to have taken on more homework as the semester ended, which made it slightly more difficult but with my last final in the books I am glad to say the semester is over. I think that this has been difficult for both the students and the professors, but everyone has been virtually helpful through zoom in order to finish the semester. I have been fortunate too for having amazing classmates that have been able to be great support throughout this spring semester."

J: "I have been filling my time with movies and great tv shows like West-world. Most of the musicians I follow on Spotify have been busy putting out singles and new albums, which has been amazing for me. I have now been able to start planting earlier and have been able to get my garden ready and seedlings planted in our sunroom."

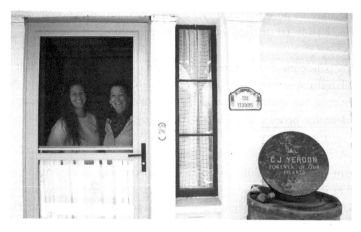

Katie + Dede Yerdon

MILFORD, NY

K: "During this time I am feeling uncertain, not knowing what the near future holds. I wonder if what was considered normal will ever be normal again in society. Personally, this has not affected me too much other than not seeing people I would see on a daily basis."

K: "My job has been very cautious during this pandemic. Luckily, I have the opportunity to work from home and few days. I am also in school, however my classes are online, so the pandemic did not affect my semester or future classes."

K: "The extra time I have throughout the day I have spent going through belongings downsizing. Being that I only have one semester left to finish my degree, I have been thinking about where I would like to adventure off and start a career. I been searching for places of employment and housing in different areas down south."

D: "My feelings during this time could be described as changing. As each day comes and goes there have been so many changes to my emotional being. So many reasons for feelings to change at any given moment. Stay positive, believe, have faith, and love myself is what I need at this moment. Personally, the effects on me, I feel so blessed to have my family and friends who are there for me when tears may flow, questions to be asked, looking for answers, just need a smile and encouraging words to help us survive whatever may come our way. My personal care for myself definitely could be better. I truly try to find the good in everything."

D: "This pandemic has affected my working world by putting not only a financial burden on me but also emotionally. I am retired from being a teacher's aide but continued my love for children by doing daycare. I also house clean for people. With social distancing I am unable to make money and enjoy the children."

D: "I am taking this time to do major downsizing in my home. I must admit I'm thankful for having this time to go through and give things away to good homes. I've been taking time to reach out to others to check in with them. Let them know I care, and we are in this together. I'm ready for some normal to return to our lives again."

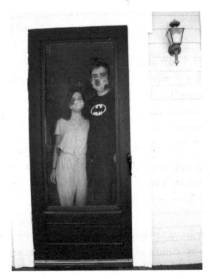

Molly Myers + Carl Loewenguth

WESTVILLE, NY

M: "I have been an emotional rollercoaster over the past few weeks. At the beginning of the quarantine, I was feeling scared and lonely from the lack of socialization, but now I feel like my emotions have become somewhat numb and I don't have a strong desire to socialize anymore. I think I have shut down a bit but have also adapted."

M: "I am so fortunate to be able to work from home. Being a fundraiser and event planner for two museums, it has certainly made my job more challenging not knowing when or how our events might go on. The money I am able to raise for the museums directly impacts the staff having jobs, so it has been very stressful trying to continue to sensitively raise money while struggling with the trauma of this crisis personally."

M: "Although I am working from home, I have also been able to work on several projects around my house as my anxiety from the COVID-19 situation was making me want to be busy all the time. I appreciate that I have had this extra time at home to paint rooms, reorganize things, and plant some seeds for veggies."

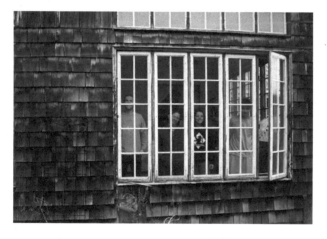

Sebastian, Kerstin, Zoe + Toby Green

MILFORD, NY

K: "I am not dealing with this very well. Although I know that we are incredibly lucky by comparison because even though we are quarantining we have space here to go outside, move, ride bikes, go for runs and walks with our dogs. We can even drive to our nearby state park and walk on the beach along a beautiful lake. Under these circumstances one would think that my mental health would be holding up, and rationally I feel as though it should. The reality is that I have been experiencing severe anxiety attacks and worsening depression since schools were closed. The saying is, a parent is only as happy as their unhappiest child, and while my children are all healthy, they are all struggling with their own issues, depression, anxiety, uncertainty, and for a mother of 5 that means my own fears are compounded fivefold. Some days the anxiety seems out of control. Sunshine helps, and the past two days have been more manageable!"

K: "I am director of a small private nursery school and kindergarten. We have been closed since Friday, March 13th. It has been very difficult trying to maintain connections with the 25 children. I immediately started a You-Tube channel and within 10 days I had uploaded 75 stories, songs, finger games and action games for the children, so that they can hear them and participate in all their favorites from home. I hold daily Zoom meetings during which we sing together, the children can chat with one another, share their favorite toys, pictures, and crafts they're working on. I read them a book every day, we play action games together and do yoga to get them moving. I think they are enjoying the routine and familiarity of the content, but I can see in their eyes that they are confused and somewhat saddened by the distance. It is very hard for me to realize that, but I think the half hour each day is better than losing the community altogether. I also zoom a few times a week with my kindergarten class, and I have been dropping off weekly work packets at these houses every Sunday evening. I have been lending my families sanitized books, puzzles, toys, and other resources from the school to help keep their children entertained at home."

K: "A couple of days ago, I was walking the dog and running through the endless list of things I could be doing, should be doing, should be glad to have time for, should be motivated to tackle, and questioning my utter inability to do anything. Then it struck me. I can't do any of those other things because I am not doing the ONE thing that I am MEANT to do. That I am made for. The one thing that energizes me, that keeps my heart pumping, makes me feel creative, purposeful, fulfilled, and that gives my life meaning. Without my children around me at Oak Hill, my days are hollow and feel meaningless. And when your days feel hollow and meaningless it's very hard to read a book, dig a garden, craft, cook, you name it. Some might think, well, all those other things would give your days meaning and purpose. Maybe so, but first I need to finish grieving the loss of all that I have spent my life building up and working on, which was there, under my nose 24/7/365 and now is gone."

Z: "I have been alternating between feeling overwhelmed and anxious and feeling positive and optimistic. Generally, the weather has a large part to play in this, as the days that I am able to be outside in the sun I feel much better and forward looking."

Z: "I lost my job at the restaurant I worked at due to COVID and the rest of my graduate school program was moved online. I finish next week, but the lack of in-person classes has taken the thrill of the end of my school career."

Z: "My finals and online classes have been filling my time. Outside of these, my brain has been exhausted and unable to focus on much else. I think that the anxiety and constant flood of news has taken up the rest of my brain power."

T: "I've been feeling less stressed with school but more stressed with being unable to leave my house. The recent weather has helped with the cabin fever."

T: "The rest of my school year was cancelled. My classes have been moved online but teachers aren't expecting as much from the students."

T: "I've been trying to pass time outside in the woods hiking and biking. When weather doesn't permit, I try to be productive and clean or something else that can improve my state of living."

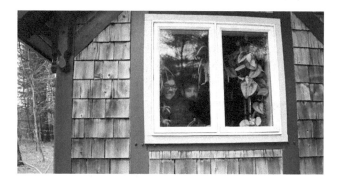

Karla Andela + Josh Simpson

MILFORD, NY

K: "I'm feeling extremely grateful that I can work from home and have a safe and loving home environment. I love being home so much, with my husband, my garden, studio, pets, and kitchen. There are days when I forget to reach out to friends and feel lonely and down about the current situation. I'm also super sad for those impacted personally by COVID-19."

K: "I am one of the few who still has a full-time job that I can do from home. It's been tough to focus sometimes, but I'm getting better about maintaining a work schedule."

K: "We definitely spend more time watching shows in the evening. I would normally feel guilty about it, but I don't! I'm baking bread—really learning the language of sourdough! I spend more time in the garden—it's a wonderful time."

J: "I've been swinging between extremely worried about humanity and the future and extremely excited about humanity and the future. I'm hopeful that this pandemic will lead to folks creating better work life balance, connect more with people they love and to think in more global terms when it comes to how we need to take care of our planet. I have also felt supremely grateful that I have the privilege of working from home."

J: "I was on partial unemployment for 3 weeks and as of 4/27/2020 my company received PPP funding and I am full time again. This pandemic has made me start to re-evaluate my life goals and I am planning on returning to college."

J: "When I was working 3 days a week, I spent the other days reading books that I have been stacking up for years now. I have also been ripping through TV shows on Netflix and Amazon Prime at a steady clip. I've also taken the time to begin preparing our second building for a massive renovation that will include the creation of Karla's pottery studio, a legit bathroom, and a hangout space for me in the upstairs."

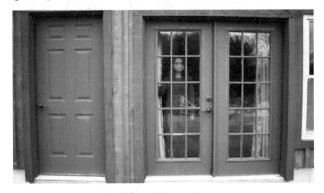

Alyx Braunius

MT. VISION, NY

A: "I've been feeling a bit anxious and trapped. I'm a homebody but also feel lonely not being able to see friends, family or being able to go anywhere. And feeling scared of not knowing what is to come."

A: "I am currently working from home and distance learning online but living somewhere where I'm not able to get internet makes that all very difficult."

A: "Even though I'm working, I have a lot of extra time not driving and getting ready for work and I do a lot more yoga, meditation, nature walks/ runs and I'm reading books for the first time in my life without it being required for school!"

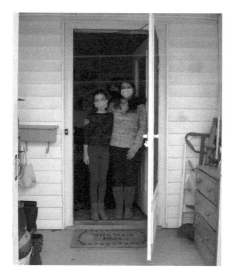

Carden, Kai + Jessica Phillips

ONEONTA, NY

C: "A little upset because I don't get to graduate from 5th and do the fun end of year things that 5th graders normally do."

C: "It makes schooling harder because we don't have teachers teaching how to do it . . . we are just expected to do work without much help."

C: "I am able to do things I don't have time to do normally. I'm also able to do fun things that I want to do, like researching hamsters and playing ukulele. I like spending more time with my animals and family. I'm happy there is Zoom and FaceTime so I can see friends."

K: "Bored, miss my friends, seems like more schoolwork than when we are in school."

K: "I don't feel like I'm learning as well as before, do not like the zoom video classrooms."

K: "Video games, walks, started working with video editing online for fun."

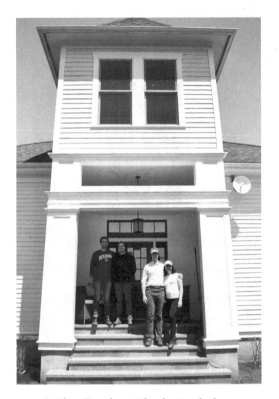

Milo Cowles, Elijah Rutledge,
Jeremey Rutledge + Melissa Sieffert

WESTVILLE, NY

J: "We have been feeling a general sadness during this time. Not only are we concerned about the spread of the virus, and the impact that it is having around the world, but we are struggling to adjust to the micro- and macrochanges everyone has had to make. Luckily, the worst thing to happen to us was our wedding being canceled. We are missing the small things like going out to eat, seeing friends and family, and making plans for the future."

J: "Our schooling has gone virtual, which has been an adjustment as many of our classes have strong discussion components that are more difficult to orchestrate via Zoom. My work as a TA has given me insight into how undergrads are dealing with the changes, and I am happy to see so much resilience in the face of great difficulty."

J: "When we are not doing schoolwork, we have been trying our hand at cooking new dishes, painting, and gardening. As the semester is coming to an end, and with the lack of usual distractions, we are finding ourselves with the time to reflect on life and ruminate on the future. We have also been talking to our families and friends much more, which has been a pleasant silver lining to the COVID-19 crisis."

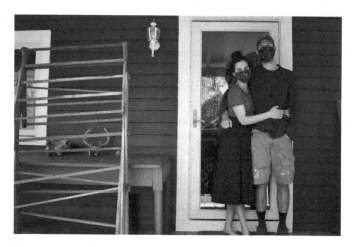

Molly Jean Feulner + Andrew Yerdon

CHERRY VALLEY, NY

M: "I have been feeling so many things during this time. Some days I feel productive at home and optimistic. Having more time to do things and not feel rushed to squeeze everything into one day is something I am grateful for during this. It is nice to have time to relax and work through this. The days are harder, I feel bombarded with information about COVID-19 and everyone else's feelings about the situation and things seem to spiral out of control quickly. I'm a major worry wart and easily fall into anxious cycles. I'm trying not to dwell on this and realize that this is temporary. I guess it's safe to say I've felt a spectrum of feelings."

M: "Andrew and I work together as contractors, and we have been able to do some small jobs outside for his mother who put her house up for sale just before the quarantine began. We haven't been able to work regularly, but with savings and not spending as much money on things like gas and going out we've been able to manage the bills so far. School transitioned to online which hasn't been hard, more disappointing honestly. For both classes it was important to be on campus and together in a classroom. I am taking Music of Film and was enjoying watching films together as a class and being able to discuss both music and film. It wasn't the same experience having this class online. My film photography class had to be switched to digital images, but this project blossomed from that, and I will be grateful to have this in the end. I hope that I gave some people a way to be a part of something during a time of isolation. Andrew and I must make a hard decision about what to do about our wedding that is planned for August. It won't be what we originally had planned."

M: "I've been trying to spend my time at home by focusing on my personal well-being mainly. We started doing Wim Hoff breathing exercises and cold showers as well as morning meditation, exercising in various ways, and trying to cook and bake more. I also love origami and have been making lots of that and considering trying to start a small business selling my pieces."

A: "During this time I am feeling a lot of things all at once it seems. The situation brings up strong emotions, both good and bad, mixed with uncertainty. I feel as though the quarantine has forced me to live and think more in the moment and I assume not knowing what the future has in store has initiated that."

A: "My job as a contractor has been affected greatly in that I have not been able to work consistently for about a month. When I can work even the simplicity of getting materials has become something stressful and that alone has deterred me from taking on work."

A: "Since I haven't been working, I've been able to fill my life with a lot of the things I truly enjoy doing as well as learning and practicing new things such as meditation. I've been practicing drums and guitar more than ever. I've been able ride Mountain Bike everyday which has been something I was only able to do before or after a full day of work or on the weekend."

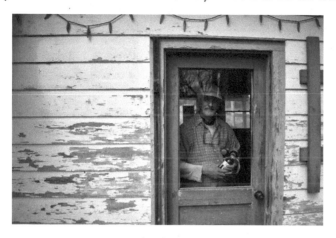

Michael Feulner

CHERRY VALLEY, NY

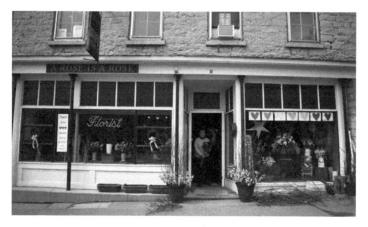

Jackie Hull (Owner of A Rose Is a Rose)

CHERRY VALLEY, NY

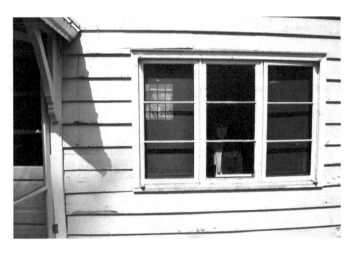

Ian Feulner

Cherry Valley, NY

I hope you all enjoy this project and continue to stay happy and healthy during this quarantine. It's hard to know what the future will hold when this is all finished, but it's easier knowing we're all in it together. Stay positive and don't forget to reach out to others for support!

—Molly Jean Feulner

Empty NYC

May 16, 2020

Joseph Suhovsky

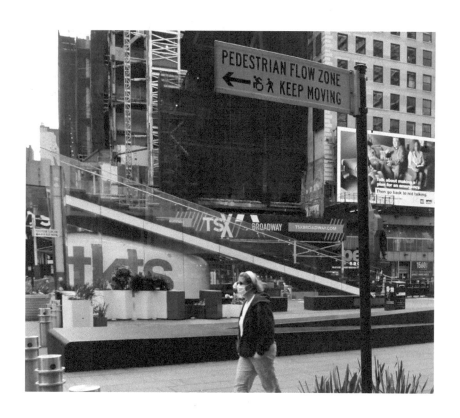

Telenovela trailer from Spanish conversation course

May 18, 2020

MARIA CRISTINA MONTOYA

Students produce a telenovela trailer as an assignment in quarantine that relates to the topic of "telenovelas mexicanas" studied in class. They re-create their feeling about the COVID-19 situation and dramatize it including the main topics of a traditional telenovela.

Problemas en Cuarentena

Cast

Morgan—Morgan Collins
Isabel's Mom—Eleanor Brown
Isabel's Dad—Jacob Yanke
Isabel—Isabel O'Brien
Alexa—Alexa Molnar
Jayda—Jayda Woodall
Joell—Joelle Zendran
Alexa's Mom—Hales Pink

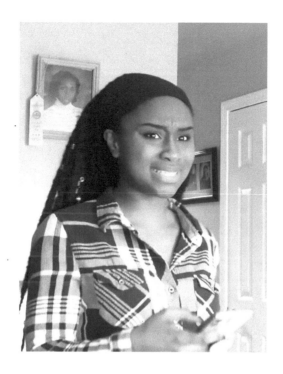

Watch Online:

View a YouTube video of Professor Maria Montoya's students' telenovela by scanning this QR Code.

Part II

Summer 2020

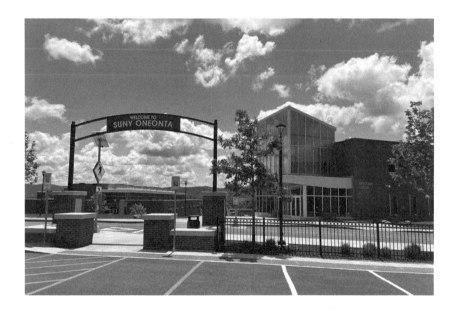

4

June 2020

SUNY ONEONTA

Campus closed. With the exception of essential personnel, faculty and staff work from home.

President Barbara Morris announces she will continue her weekly, virtual updates for faculty and staff.

ONEONTA

June 3—Otsego County Board of Representatives continues with COVID budget cuts, including a spending freeze.

June 15—Governor Cuomo allows public buildings to open in the City of Oneonta with 50 percent capacity.

June 22—Bassett Healthcare partially lifts hospital visitor restrictions.

NEW YORK

June 15—New York City begins to reopen, allowing outdoor dining and some businesses such as hair salons and barber shops to admit a limited number of customers.

USA

June 10—Cases of COVID-19 in the United States reach 2 million.

June 19—The United States reported more than 30,000 new infections.

WORLD

June 11—The number of COVID-19 cases in Africa topped 200,000.

Protesting in the Age of the Pandemic

June 7, 2020

MATTHEW C. HENDLEY

It seems obvious in retrospect that history does not stand still even during a biological emergency. Long simmering problems like racial discrimination and racial inequality do not go away when plague stalks the land. Police brutality does not cease. Injustice does not take a break. However, it does lead to an important question:

How does one protest during a pandemic?

I suppose the answer comes in two words: Purposefully and carefully

My family decided to join the Black Lives Matter protest planned in front of the Otsego County Court House in Cooperstown, New York on June 7, 2020. Our children insisted that we go. As we are a biracial family this cause was not abstract to us. It was real. We made signs together including one that said "Black Lives Matter," which included the faces of people of color whose lives were ended far too soon by white violence—Breonna Taylor, George Floyd, Emmett Till and Ahmaud Arbery.

Our family all wore masks. We all waved our signs and felt a sense of unity with everyone gathered. There were 500 people standing in the sunshine holding signs, but they kept socially distant. On that beautiful summer's day in an idyllic setting of the place that is called "America's perfect village," speeches invoked the ugly underbelly of America—its historic record of racism. Just steps from the lovely old inns and shimmering waters of "Glimmerglass Lake," we heard Lee Fisher, the head of the local NAACP speak about systemic racism. We heard Shannon McHugh, a member of the

Oneonta Commission on Community Relations and Human Rights instruct the crowd on how white people can be allies and what they should do. We heard Rev. La Dana Clark point to the links of religion and protest. We heard Bryce Wooden, a longtime Oneonta resident who is biracial, speak of when the police burst into his home when he was a young boy in a mistaken drug raid. The speakers were powerful. The crowd was enthusiastic and peaceful. The sun shone with a gentle breeze. We left emboldened with a new sense of purpose and were glad that we experienced it as a family.

There was a deep irony at work as we protested during the pandemic. Social distance and masks were used by the protesters as a conscious way to avoid the contagion of COVID. However, the point of the protest was that the contagion of racism cannot be so easily controlled. It has been long lasting, deadly and there is no easy cure. No masks and no vaccines will protect you from it. Nevertheless, we did leave the protest with a sense of hope. We signed up to join the local NAACP and gave a donation and prepared to think about how America could be better.

There would be other local protests that summer. Our daughter attended one downtown. Michelle and I went to Neahwa Park to celebrate Juneteenth (marking the formal end of slavery) with a candlelight vigil and listened

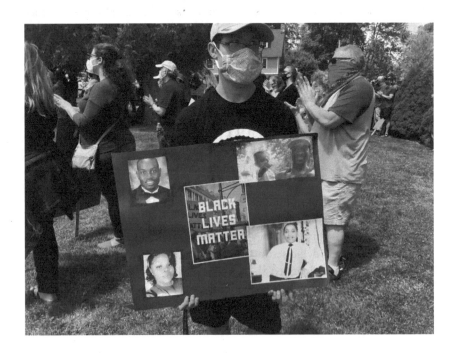

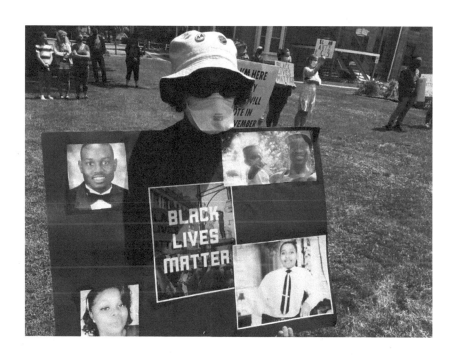

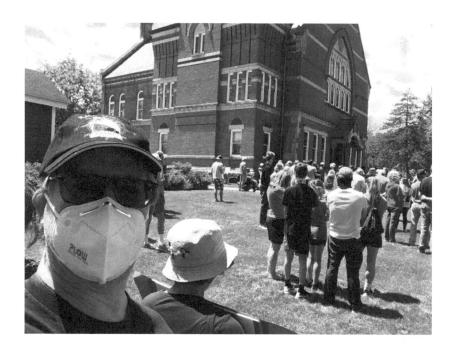

on a summer's evening to local speakers. All these events were masked and socially distant. They all mattered.

Still, I think the day together as a family in Cooperstown was the most memorable for us. Together we gathered with many others during a pandemic on a brilliant sunny day. We were passionate and peaceful. Purposeful and receptive. It was a way to acknowledge that change might still be possible. Biological diseases are caused by nature and spread by people. Racial hatred is fanned by people and spread by people. If a nation can come together to conquer one, why can't they conquer the other as well?

3 months after quarantine
June 10, 2020

Maria Cristina Montoya

I decided to try make up again today, June 6th. For a moment I couldn't remember the order, the brushes, and the colors I used, before leaving for class. I miss my office at Schumacher. I miss my classroom. I miss my practice.

Zoom—a new household term

June 15, 2020

Carolyn Leon-Palm

Before March 16, I had not heard of Zoom, but since then, it has become a word we use frequently in our household. Between my daughter's Zoom classes for school and dance, my Zoom meetings for work, and my husband joining in Zoom calls with friends and family, we are all too familiar with it. It just strikes me that something I didn't think of pre-pandemic or a term I even referred to, is so common now. I even find myself thinking after a Zoom call with friends in other states or countries, "Why didn't we do this before?" Sure, we were all busier and didn't need to think of ways to stay in touch virtually like we have had to do in quarantine. However, I am now finding it a fun way of having a group gathering with distant friends and family and bringing people together. Since being in quarantine, there is a group of us who went to college together in Ohio, who now Zoom once a month and have reconnected after 20 years! Some live in Canada, Florida, etc. but for that hour each month, it is like we are all sitting around in someone's living room sharing stories, laughs and our feelings about quarantine. I know for some, having to have Zoom meetings and Zoom classes may not be something that brings up such positive thoughts, but there is this other aspect to Zoom which has made quarantine in our household more bearable.

5

July 2020

SUNY ONEONTA

July 9—It is announced that the Theater Department is making PPE to help front-line workers.

ONEONTA

July 4—The Hometown Fourth of July festival is canceled.

NEW YORK

July 22—Ten more states have been added to the travel advisory, bringing the total to thirty-one.

USA

July 10—A new milestone is reached: 68,000 new cases a day, a single-day record.

July 31—New infections reported for the month of July alone reached 1.9 million, nearly 42 percent of all the cases reported since the pandemic began.

WORLD

July 17—India reached 1 million cases of COVID-19.

Hindsight 2020

July 8, 2020

Maggie McCann

Looking back at my diary entries from the beginning of the pandemic [March 25, 2020, March 28, 2020]. There's a lot I'd like to comment on now that I'm looking back on it:

There's so much about this I can't even believe I wrote looking back, there were so many things I was going to have to worry about besides the variety of clothes I had at home, people were literally dying by the thousands and my biggest concern was my wardrobe, that mind-set changed pretty quickly. Also, this was the last time I saw Ryan in person for another two and a half months, even writing that I never could've imagined we'd be three and a half months in and still where we are. No one could have predicted this.

Friday Takeout Unmasked

July 14, 2020

MICHELLE HENDLEY

My family started a new tradition shortly after the Governor declared a state of emergency in New York. To support our local businesses, break the monotony of being at home all day, avoid preparing dinner, consume delicious food, and establish an event to look forward to, we decided to order from a different restaurant on Fridays. At this point of the pandemic, we were instructed to stay home and social distance. COVID-19 cases and hospitalizations were increasing at an alarming rate in New York City. Cases were confirmed in Otsego County. Consequently, we ordered our food online and requested contact-less delivery. One of the first restaurants we ordered from serves Jamaican-American food. It was slated to have its grand opening on the day the Governor ordered businesses to close. Luckily for us as connoisseurs of Jamaican food, the owners decided to transition to the take-out model. When the owner delivered the food to the house, I was on my front porch. She and I maintained a distance of at least six feet as she gently rested our food at the top of the stairs to my porch. She was grateful for the business, and I was grateful for the delicious food.

We continued this pattern of contact-free delivery of our Friday meal until early May when we saw signs that the COVID-19 situation was improving. At this point in the pandemic, COVID-19 hospitalization and death rates were slowing down in New York. We were now required to wear masks in public when social distancing was impossible. Our next-

170

door neighbor had closed his Japanese restaurant in March and promised to open only when he felt the pandemic was under control. We were happy when he announced in late April that he was reopening his restaurant for takeout. To celebrate the opening of our neighbor's restaurant, we decided to order our Friday meal from him. We were feeling braver and decided to venture to the restaurant and pick up our food order. We walked to the restaurant. We wore our masks. We picked up our food from our neighbor. He met all the customers at the front door. He was thrilled to see us. He wore a mask and gloves. He placed hand sanitizer on the pick-up table for his customers. He prominently displayed a sign about the benefits of wearing masks and good hygiene. He gave us our food. We returned home and enjoyed our delicious meal.

We continued our Friday tradition into June. On one Friday, as our region entered phase three of reopening, we became even bolder. We decided to order from a restaurant we had never previously ordered from or dined at in pre-pandemic days. We had heard good things about it. We followed the usual pattern: order online, go to the restaurant, wear mask, get food. As I approached the restaurant, I noticed a sign on the door indicating that customers entering the restaurant must wear masks. No problem. We were wearing our masks. We entered the building. There were two staff and one customer in the restaurant. Ironically, none of them was wearing a mask. I greeted the staff. The person behind the bar looked uncomfortable and confused. "May I help you?" he asked. The question was distinctly unfriendly. "I am here to pick up my food order," I said in a friendly and polite manner. My response appeared to confuse him even more. "What did you order?" I told him. More confusion. What was the problem? My mask? The sign on the door specifically stated that anyone entering the restaurant must wear a mask. I was wearing a plain white mask this evening, not the other one I kept at home that declared my allegiance to the Toronto Raptors. Was it my brown skin? My curly black hair? My brightly colored dress? One of my daughter's health care providers once informed me that the yellow fleece I was wearing was "rather bright" and the comment was not meant to be complimentary. Was it because I was not a regular? Was it my Canadian accent which still has traces of a Jamaican inflection that he could not quite place? Many years ago, a SUNY Oneonta faculty member once asked me if I was from Long Island. I thought that was an odd question, but I digress. Did the man behind the counter think I was a fugitive from downstate? An outsider? Still looking dubious, he moved to the kitchen to ask the chef about my order. The chef emerged from the kitchen with the meals I had ordered and passed them on to the waitress. She started fiddling with the cash register. "I already paid," I said, keeping my tone even and still friendly. My husband tried to make small talk with her, but his attempts did not break the tension in the room. The waitress confirmed my payment, gave us our food, and we left.

"Is it just me, or was that really uncomfortable?" I asked my husband when we were safely in our car. "Nope," he replied, "That was definitely unwelcoming." "It's a good thing you were with me," I responded. Once an outsider, always an outsider, despite living in Oneonta for almost twenty years, I thought to myself. Well, at least we had our food, though unfortunately it turned out to be like the service, unpleasant. "Next week, we ought to order dinner from the Indian restaurant," my husband suggested. "Yes," I agreed. The food is delicious, the staff is friendly, and they wear their masks.

The time my kid took her mask off at Target

July 15, 2020

Melissa Marietta

I may go viral soon.

Recently, my husband and two daughters stopped by Target to pick up a few odds and ends. Throughout quarantine, my kids have been earning money and their pockets were burning. They both thought carefully about what to buy, giving me a quiet satisfaction that, at 9 and 13, they are beginning to understand budgeting and the cost of the objects of their desire. My 9-year-old, Charlotte, was quick to make her selections: a weird stuffed animal thing in a plastic box shaped like a melting popsicle, sharpies for drawing class, and stickers.

As usual, my 13-year-old cemented herself in the office supply aisle. Caroline is a collector, having accumulated over 50 notebooks and a dozen or more water bottles. Mechanical pencils are a newer passion, and she requests them daily. She is so passionate about her collectibles that she often gets stuck on only one topic that she can't unstick herself from thinking about. Right now, it is pencils. "Mom, will you buy me mechanical pencils? Can we go to the store to buy them? Can you order them on Amazon? Can you do it now?"

Having her own money helps Caroline understand that we can buy what we'd like with money we've earned. It also helps her practice strengthening her impulse control, gain a sense of delayed gratification, and improve her math skills. As a kiddo with a developmental delay, these are all really critical milestones. Sometimes Caroline's behavior is like that of a small child, which is frustrating to all of us in her family because we have expectations for the behavior and actions of children as they age. Life would sure be easier if Caroline had the competencies and maturity of other kids her age, but she doesn't, so we continue to navigate the bumps in the road.

While she was still hovering over the pencils, I stood at the end of the aisle and gave Caroline a five-minute warning, a technique we use often to help her transition between activities. Dancing a bit between aisles in an attempt to keep 6 feet of distance between me and the other shoppers, I then prompted Caroline with a one-minute countdown, and she reluctantly turned toward me with a small pack of mechanical pencils in her hand. Following a protocol we established with her behavior specialist, I praised her for making a choice and transitioning without any issues.

"All set, buddy?" I asked her, sensing her frustration at being pushed to make a decision not at her own pace.

"Yeah. I guess so. I'll just get these today." I could tell she was internally processing all the things we've been working on teaching her, and I was proud. Just a few years ago, we weren't able to leave a Target without her tantrumming over being told no to a purchase request. Now, she can bring her own money, prioritize her purchases, and leave happy with her decision.

My husband and I checked out first, spending too much money on not very much, like underwear and shampoo, but also scoring a few containers of that amazing Target trail mix with chocolate. Charlotte was next and I pumped sanitizer onto her hands as she stepped away from the checkout area. Finally, Caroline placed her pack of pencils on the conveyor belt. She methodically and cautiously pulled the money from her wallet and gathered her small bag with a satisfied smile. I pumped sanitizer onto her hands as we left.

I walked slightly ahead of Caroline, who moves at a slower pace. My mind was on dinner plans and getting home before anything frozen thawed on this hot summer day. I stopped to look both ways before stepping off of the sidewalk and heard someone shouting. A young woman passed me and Caroline. She made eye contact with me, and I'd tried to eye smile at her, as I'm now practicing since nobody can see my mouth behind my mask. Now, I realized she was shouting at me. Or rather at Caroline who had just taken off her mask. "Put on your mask! What's wrong with you!" I turned toward the woman as her words lashed in our direction and echoed across the parking lot. A few passersby had stopped to watch the interaction. The young woman, two dozen paces from us, stood firm, her feet planted in a power stance, her arms waving, and her eyes blazing above her mask. "There's a pandemic happening! Put on a mask! What is wrong with people?"

Disinterested in escalating the situation and concerned for Caroline, I grabbed her hand, put my head down, and walked swiftly toward the car. My masked face was hot and turning red. I was so embarrassed. Caroline started crying. As we drove home, I wondered if that woman had taken a photo of us. I couldn't recall if she had her device in hand. Were Caroline and I about to go viral? Would the world soon see me as just another angry Karen, pushing her privileged agenda over the safety of others?

We barely left the house for three months; we still wear masks and we socially distance. Asking if the kids have their masks and sanitizer is now as routine as reminding them to go to the bathroom before we leave. I'm frustrated when I see people in public not wearing a mask or wearing it tucked under their nose. To the woman I encountered yesterday at Target, I am sorry, and I apologize for not doing my job as a parent by ensuring my child followed masking protocol. I should have been walking alongside her and caught her unmasking. I know you are upset and scared and maybe someone you know, or love has been a victim of COVID and all you wanted to do was go to Target and buy underwear and trail mix without worrying you'd be infected because of some stupid Karen and her kid. We learned our lesson and, next time we go out, we will do better.

If I had the chance to meet her, I would share Caroline's story with her and tell her how proud we are to have her as our daughter and watch her overcome things, like her ability to wear a mask despite her sensory challenges. I would apologize. If she were still listening, I'd challenge her. I'd ask her if she had ever been shamed as a child when she made a mistake and I'd ask her how she felt at that moment. I'd ask if it changed her behavior and I'd ask her if she carried that shame long after it took place, having forgotten what action precipitated the shaming, but not the feeling of being told you are less than.

It was a teachable moment for me. It reminded me that our actions speak loudly and make a lasting impact, for better and worse.

6

August 2020

SUNY ONEONTA

August 24—Classes begin at SUNY Oneonta.

August 28—SUNY President Barbara Jean Morris and SUNY Chancellor Jim Malatras announce a two-week pause on campus activities due to rising COVID numbers.

August 30—On-campus classes put on pause for at least two weeks at SUNY Oneonta.

August 31—New York State deploys team to SUNY Oneonta to assist with testing and tracing efforts.

ONEONTA

August 31—COVID task force with City of Oneonta, state officials, and SUNY Oneonta administrators meet to deal with ongoing crisis at SUNY Oneonta.

NEW YORK

August 7—Governor Cuomo announces schools will reopen to in-person instruction at the start of the school year with students wearing masks.

August 24—Governor Cuomo announces high school sports classified as lower risk (including soccer, tennis, field hockey, and swimming) will be able to resume practice and play starting on September 21, with restrictions.

August 25—Gyms, museums, and aquariums began reopening on August 24 at 25 percent capacity with mask requirement.

USA

August 11—Trump administration reaches deal with Moderna—will pay $1.5 billion for 100 million doses.

August 15—FDA approves saliva test.

August 17—COVID-19 now the third leading cause of death in the US.

WORLD

August 3—In the UK, the monthlong "Eat Out to Help Out" scheme begins, offering a 50 percent discount on meals at indoor venues, three days per week, with the remainder of the cost picked up by the British government. Over 160 million meals were consumed at cost to government of £849 million.

August 7—WHO published updated guidance on public health surveillance for COVID-19, with clearer definitions on suspected and probable cases.

Soccer in the age of COVID-19

August 10, 2020

Miguel León

One of the many things we have lost in these pandemic times is to be close to our friends. We miss shaking hands, having lengthy intellectual conversations face to face or playing group sports. We are afraid of the virus, and this keeps us apart. We are afraid of being infected and getting sick. After more than four months of the COVID-19 outbreak, we know a great deal about this virus, thanks to the studies of competent scientists. For example, we know that this virus gets transmitted from one person to another when in close contact for an extended period of time. For that reason, health authorities recommend social distancing, wearing a mask and avoiding being in closed spaces to minimize infection. With that in mind, I suggested to my friend Matthew that we play some "socially distant" soccer. In other words, pass the ball around with each player far enough (30 meters) from each other and do that for 45 minutes or so every Saturday in Neahwa Park. The weather is being very cooperative. We have enjoyed beautiful sunny days. We agreed on avoiding using our hands when we manipulate the soccer ball, and only use our feet to kick the ball. If we need to communicate, we have to speak a bit louder. We won't do "high fives" and when it is time to end the exercise we will depart individually. We discovered that this was a nice workout. We will keep doing it as weather permits and until this pandemic ends.

We Used to Wait:
Or Rediscovering the Lost Art of
Letter Writing in the Great Pandemic of 2020

August 10, 2020

Matthew C. Hendley

It figures that Arcade Fire, a band from Montreal, would speak to my current frame of mind. In their recent song "We Used to Wait," they point to the angst of being in the current social media culture and contrast it with the world of letters sent through the post. I am a dual citizen of Canada and the USA who did graduate study in Montreal and am living through the great pandemic of 2020. What I have been thinking about is this: In our new world of instant connectivity and constant social media interaction, have we lost something vital that helped past generations survive similar uncertainties—the venerable art of letter writing?

I must admit I have always been old-fashioned about letter writing. To this day, I still like getting mail. I subscribe to print magazines. Every year I send out an actual hard copy Christmas newsletter and Christmas cards. Perhaps I am a dinosaur. I have fond memories of getting mail from American grandparents when I was a child growing up in Canada, of receiving notes and letters from my parents when I was living away from home as an undergraduate and sending and receiving countless letters to my future wife when we lived in separate cities during undergraduate summers and graduate school (as well as research trips). In the day—I loved getting postcards too.

There would be a professional photo on the front of the card with exotic stamps and a cheery scrawl on the back of the card outlining whatever foreign adventure the sender was on. I always got a kick out of picking up letters from the mailbox, sorting through them and opening them. Letters are so tangible and personal. There is something special when you realize that a person has taken the time to compose some ordered thoughts on a piece of paper by hand and send them your way. Better still, you can read them at leisure. If the letter is long you can even read it in segments and re-read it. If the letter is meaningful, you can keep it for years.

Which brings me to my two points—Why have we lost the art of letter writing and can the pandemic offer a chance at a revival? I suppose no one writes letters anymore because it takes too long and seems to be too much effort. Better to send a GIF, make a post, send an emoji, or tap out a few words on Facebook to "Stay in touch." However, I would hazard to say that this does not really fill people's hunger for connection. Social media's greatest advantages are the ability to send images and quick succinct (hopefully witty) sentences and phrases. It cannot be denied that the ability to chronicle one's trips, days, adventures by pictures sent from mobile phones through Instagram or other apps as well as putting on Facebook gives a sense of immediacy. What I worry about though is that people cannot dig as deep when they have a character limit on Twitter or messaging services. Let's also admit that there is not often too much contemplation put into most instant communication. The point is not to choose your words carefully but to send them quickly. It gives a dopamine hit to the brain to send and receive such things. Reflection is usually absent. People are busy and the technology exists, so it is used. It all makes sense. However, as Arcade Fire's words point out—it has also created enormous anxiety over what people are missing or what others are up to. Maybe no one sleeps at night anymore.

Letter writing is something different. It is almost a form of meditation. By getting out a blank piece of paper you can craft your own tale and tell your own narrative. Events, observations, thoughts over the past few weeks (or months if it has been a while) can flow out of your pen. Inner thoughts not always best shared through social media (which might be reposted to others) can also be revealed. Due to the pandemic, I have not been able to travel to see family in Canada or friends more distant in places like the UK. I have taken my own advice and begun to rediscover letter writing. I took a deep breath, got out some pieces of lined paper and started. I found it very rewarding. Sitting down for 45 minutes to an hour and just writing out my thoughts made me feel more focused and more connected. I was able to explain to myself as I explained to others the meaning of what I have been experiencing through the pandemic. I was able to shape my thoughts and put them into a narrative. It felt personal. It felt real. I felt more relaxed and calmer. When it was done it felt concrete. I put it into an envelope—sealed it up and then had an excuse to get outside and walk to a mailbox. Then (again as Arcade Fire sang) I waited until it was received. Inevitably the recipients got back to me in more modern ways through email or telephone conversations. However, they were as pleasantly surprised to get an 8-page handwritten letter as I was to send it. My mother complimented my letter as "newsy" which is a nice way to put it. I will see if my recipients are inspired enough to write me back but that is beside the point. The art of composing and writing letters was invigorating and I will repeat it. Though they are not always happy about it I have even conscripted my children into writing much shorter letters to their relatives as well.

As a historian I have read and continue to read countless letters from the past. In British archives, I have seen the indecipherable handwriting of Lord Curzon (one-time Viceroy of India). I have read over the letters of other early 20th century worthies like Lord Roberts and Lord and Lady Milner. I have sat in the home of the descendants of female aristocratic leaders like Lady Forster and read her words retrieved from a trunk in the basement of their home. I have held letters written and signed by British Prime Ministers Winston Churchill and Harold Macmillan. I have sat in Hong Kong and read the letters and correspondence of past governors like Sir Murray MacLehose. When I wrote an article about the Shakespeare Tercentenary of 1916, I did research in the National Archives in Washington, DC and read letters by President Wilson. There is something enthralling about holding the correspondence of long dead figures you are studying. They literally spring to life out of the page. I have no illusions that I will have any long-term historical importance myself. However, in a small way by reviving letter writing on my own I feel I am keeping the record going as well as reaching out to people I care about. Letter writing is both therapeutic and meaningful to me. Maybe others may rediscover it too.

The View from Here

August 12, 2020

SVEN ANDERSON

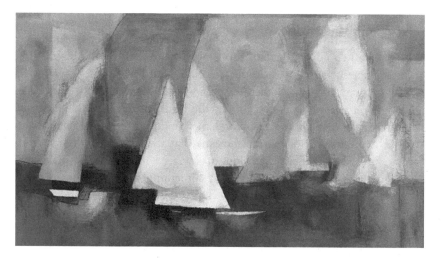

Regatta, 2020

I had great plans, but then again, I always have great plans. Finish off this semester, do a quick spin around a summer class and then I was on sabbatical for the rest of 2020. Not due back at school until mid-January. I was going to Iceland, Scandinavia, along with Canada and Alaska, in an attempt to get a photograph of the ever-elusive aurora borealis. The Canada/ Alaska portion was to be travelled via a nicely rigged out van-sized RV. Then something else happened. I guess I should have known, it was inevitable. You see, my artwork is based on Free Association. So, when I work, if I cross something in my path, I abandon my current path and take off on the new one, until another one crosses my path. This way I always end up in some place new. So, when the coronavirus decided to cross my path, I should not have been surprised. All of a sudden, my sabbatical dreams of a trip imagined for several years were lying in a pile of cancelled reservations. As my ability to walk is diminishing faster than the Trump presidency, the window of opportunity for me to take these trips is getting smaller. With a disease that affects the lungs, I am a prime example of someone who needs to avoid the virus at all costs. This means I sit in a chair at home. The pandemic has given me plenty of time to sit. Sit and think and sit and stare. Being compulsive, I count things, how many windowpanes, how many wood strips are in the ceiling. Every day, the count never changes. Mostly I stare out the window and watch the birds on our feeders. We started out in the Spring with over a dozen feeders hanging outside our windows, but a visit from a huge black bear made us rethink that idea. Now we hang just a few and bring them in every night. In the morning, the goldfinches remind us "It's time" to put out the feeders. Thank God for the birds.

So, you could say that my sabbatical has gone to the birds, but after all, that's not such a bad place to be. Feeling confined, I was looking for a subject to draw, or paint, something that was readily available. I decided to embark on a series of paintings about the birds on my feeders. Not really wanting to create a photorealistic or James Audubon likeness, I wanted to try and come up with an abstract means that would convey the idea of a bird and everything about them into an image. I made a series of sketches of my visitors, thinking I would glean something from these images that would give me an idea. But soon my mind started to wander, and I found myself surfing the interwebs, checking up on what my friends were doing and seeing if the world had crumbled yet. I came upon a post from a friend who is heavily into sailing and read of their adventures in a race on Lake Huron and Lake Michigan. The post included a simple picture taken from their boat with nothing but part of the boat and endless water ahead. But the story was enough to get my mind out of my stagnant room and out onto the water. I imagined the regatta of sailboats, dancing on the wind and I was gone. I was no longer stuck in my house; I could feel the wind and the spray. Thank God I wasn't actually in a boat, or I would have been puking my guts out as I am incredibly motion sick enabled. I spent the afternoon drawing sailboats, and the result is posted above. Like paintings of the old masters, where they have x-rayed the painting to discover other previous images buried beneath, to get a glimpse of the artist's process. If you would just look at the original Photoshop file, I used to lay out the image before taking it to my paint synthesis program, you would see, the bottom couple layers are all sketches of birds on my feeders. As the layers were added, the birds disappeared, and sailboats emerged. I'm still drawing birds, but I don't know if I can share them, it's kind of like posting pictures of your kids on social media. They are still a little too close. Throughout the pandemic, I have been sketching every day, and every day I start out with a perfectly good plan but *Along Comes Mary* (see how I worked that reference to "The Association" into this, they were a singing group from the '60s for you young punks) and I'm off on something completely different. I've not finished a plan yet, and plan not to.

Staying Centered: My Baseball Chat Group

August 13, 2020

BILL SIMONS

The Coronavirus Era is far from over. The SUNY community has demonstrated dedication in preparing for distance learning. With restrictions and new responsibilities, we have all found our internal gyroscopes challenged. United University Professions (UUP) members have shared accounts of activities, including pet bonding, special recipes, gardening, singing, and photography, that keep them centered. Here's mine: a baseball chat group.

Chat group membership has fluctuated, but our current roster lists 26, the same number of players carried by a major league team. We communicate by email list serv. Our bond is an enduring love of baseball. All of us have prior history with at least some of the others. One of the connections is participation in the Cooperstown Symposium on Baseball and American Culture. The latter association means that a core of us have also played together in spirited town ball games. Although MLB has belatedly started play in an anticipated 60-game season, the reality is that baseball in the U.S. from Little League to the minor leagues has, by and large, left the playing field. From the convening of pitchers and catchers in February until autumn chill announces the final game of World Series, we usually find balance in our lives from the rhythms of the game. Hence, as a substitute, during the late winter our baseball chat emerged—and, despite the return of MLB, still carries on.

Mark is the founder of the group, initially presented as a platform for baseball trivia questions. Although that continues, the network has come to also include sharing of information, video and text links, well-told stories, witticism, debate challenges, selection of all-time ethnic all-star teams, proposals for reforming baseball, nostalgia—and eloquent digression. Structure, of sorts, evolved with the appointment of David as the Commissioner. David also carries the sobriquet of "The Batboy," earned by serving in that capacity for the St. Louis Cardinals during the prime of Curt Flood and Lou Brock.

No day passes without robust chat group communication, and some days bring a lot of it. Baseball trivia questions still form the spine of the back-and-forth. Although there might be a couple of strikes—or more—before a correct answer emerges, a winning response will invariably come. Protocols preclude Googling for an answer or consulting a baseball reference book: such a breach might, if discovered, lead to the suspension of the miscreant by the Commissioner. In terms of baseball IQ, this is a very erudite group, whose membership, through the years, has published books and articles about what we still stubbornly claim is our national pastime. As the passage of the baseball seasons attest, we are not a young group, but we are still passionate.

We also do virtual celebrations and did so on May 6th to honor the 89th birthday of Willie Mays, the Giants' legendary centerfielder and arguably the greatest living ballplayer. Amongst the stories told on that special day was the following, perhaps apocryphal: "Willie went in to see Giants owner Horace Stoneham to get a raise. Stoneham refused. Departing, Willie instead of turning left to go home, turned right. Willie went to the local Chevrolet dealership, bought a car, told the salesman to bill the car to the Giants, and then went home." Our devotion to baseball—and need for a baseball chat forum during the battle against the coronavirus—will continue during our online teaching semester.

For many of us, the love of the game came early. My sister recently rediscovered and forwarded an old family film of me, aged 7, swinging at baseballs. Nearly 65-years later on these shuttered corona days, I daily hit baseballs into a backyard net, a vignette I shared with my baseball chat group.

Pandemic Vacation

August 15, 2020

MATTHEW C. HENDLEY

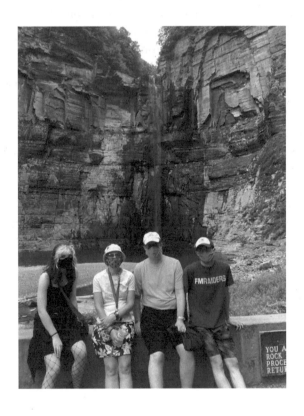

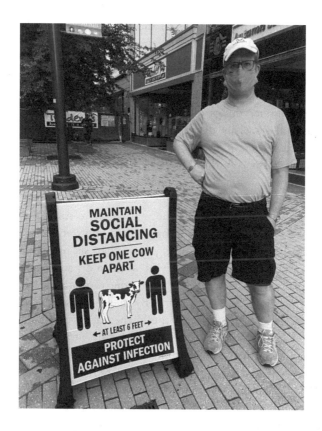

Can you go on a family vacation during a global pandemic?

With proper planning, suitable paranoia, and limited expectations, the answer is yes. What follows is a short description of the efforts of our family for a getaway during the pandemic summer of 2020. My tale shows that sometimes with a bit of planning, attention to safety, and flexibility, you can still have a bit of joy in the grimmest of times.

At first, I thought the suggestion was insane: "Can we please go on a family vacation?" The question came from my son Jon, who is on the autism spectrum and can get very focused on matters that are important to him. During the peak of the COVID pandemic in Spring 2020 this idea seemed extremely unlikely. With the spike of COVID cases in New York in the Spring, vacationing was the last thing on my mind. During the worst of the Spring COVID surge, my life revolved around teaching all my classes online and nervously venturing out to the grocery store once a week. I did not go to restaurants. I did not socialize with friends. I did not go into my office except briefly some evenings to grab some books or documents. No friends entered our house. It was like being in a siege (or in a prison) with my family as my only real social contacts. The highlight of the week was Friday night takeout for supper.

By the summer things did improve a bit. Cases dropped. We kept on our masks and socially distanced ourselves from non-family members. We still abided by our rule of having no friends in the house. However, we began to have socially distant social gatherings of a few select friends on our front porch. We had a stone patio put in our backyard and started tentatively to host a few select friends there. We ordered takeout and ate it all outside. We felt slightly more normal but were still quite careful. No shared cutlery! No shared drinks! Tons of hand sanitizers! Face masks when you are not eating! Everyone is sitting more than six feet apart! By June I began to go into my office a few days a week to do academic work there.

By the time late July rolled around, the vacation idea could not be avoided. Jon persisted. He had a point. By then he was even working a few days a week (masked of course) in the kitchen at Applebee's as a summer job. He felt a family vacation was a sacred family ritual. I relented.

We had cancelled a huge summer trip to Canada for 2020. We were going to visit our much-loved family in Ontario and then fly out to Newfoundland, Canada's easternmost province. I had never been to New-foundland (fondly called "The Rock" by Newfoundlanders). It was the first part of North America visited by Europeans (by the Vikings in the 11th century and John Cabot in the 15th century). It was the last province to join Canada in 1949. It had its own distinct dialect of English, its own extremely potent brand of rum (called Screech), a long history associated with the fisheries and shipping and distinct wooden architecture around the scenic harbor of St. John's. It had history, scenery, whale, and puffin watching tours. Ocean vistas and views beckoned. COVID shattered our Newfoundland plans. We could not cross the border. We did not feel safe undertaking a long vacation. So, we scaled back our expectations.

We settled on Ithaca, New York. I nervously booked a hotel near Cornell University for only 2 nights. We planned it out so we would eat picnics outside or at restaurants with outdoor dining. My expectations were immediately exceeded when we stopped at Whitney Point (which we had driven through dozens of times on the way to Canada without it registering in my consciousness at all) and found a beautiful park by a lake for a picnic lunch. Upon arrival in Ithaca, we nervously checked into our hotel. We brought wipes to wipe down our hotel room. We wore masks. We got the take-out breakfast from the hotel and ate our muffins on a nearby picnic bench.

While in Ithaca we did not do too much yet it was such a pleasant change from our isolated lives in Oneonta. We went to several beautiful parks and hiked to see waterfalls. We walked around Cornell University. I read a trashy novel in the evenings. In honor of our vegetarian daughter Sara, we ate a great all vegetarian meal at tables outside of the famous Moosewood restaurant. We walked around the Ithaca Commons pedestrian area. We got ice creams. We tried to go swimming at a park at Cayuga Lake, but it rained. It was ordinary. But it was extraordinary. Even with masks, hand sanitizers, a bit of paranoia about keeping socially distant from strangers and no indoor dining or museums, it was great. It was wonderful to break routine and explore even for a bit. We felt rejuvenated. We stayed healthy. All went well.

In the months to come, especially when COVID's next wave hit with a resurgence in the Fall, I kept telling my ever-patient wife Michelle, "You know, Jon was right about that summer vacation!" At least we created one pleasant memory from the horrible season of COVID.

Where did I leave off?

August 21, 2020

MARIA CRISTINA MONTOYA

Oh, yes, I was taking hikes with Shiro, my dog, up the South-side hill. This quarantine activity stopped right after we almost got EATEN by a Coyote in the middle of the day. However, that story is too long and dramatic to record it for Pandemic History. We escaped unhurt yet traumatized, and I ended up loving my dog even more.

I continued walking South-side drive up and down, taught my regular summer courses, and tried to disconnect from reality. This is easy for some of us that live on the mountain. In July I felt nostalgic for my classroom. It has been the longest summer break at home with my family. Listened to U.S. news through the lens of Colombian news and did not want to think.

Like our students, two days before the deadline, I am not totally ready, but see the light.

The light of a computer screen and multiple faces, pictures, or initials. One part of me feels excited for what is ahead, a new way of teaching and learning; another part of me feels worried and misses student contact. I drove by a live campus two days ago, calmer, organized, and full of young minds.

I guess I am ready for my online full-planned experience, just need to pick up my office.

See you in TEAMS.

The light at the end of the Tunnel: A COVID-19 experience

August 22, 2020

JOHNATHON SHANNON

Dear Diary,

COVID-19 has changed my life in many ways and has altered my life and most likely the course of history through changing my impact and everyone else's impact on the world. I say this because no matter how small, everyone's actions impact others and the world in some shape and form. COVID-19 has made me change many things about my life and has caused drastic changes in which I had no control over. I am not sure whether I am better off now or before the virus due to these changes, some being positive and some negative. Along with the entire world, in some areas COVID-19 has proved to be a nightmare for me and my family and made many experiences far less than pleasant and in turn has negatively impacted my life and my family's life. However, in other areas COVID-19 has helped me and my family and has positively impacted me and my family. As a whole though, the impact of COVID-19 on me and my family has been far more negative than positive. In the spring of 2020, I experienced the loss of friends and my boxing family, and this has caused emotional pain which has yet to fully pass.

The journey through COVID-19 has been emotionally painful for me. Waking up one day to find out that you would never see your friends and teachers again was my reality. The sorrow of realizing that you can never experience a true end to High School is devastating. I will never forget when my entire school switched to online learning, and I was provided with a false sense of security that school would resume in April. Then, in a flash that hope was blown away, only to reveal the ugly truth that it was over, there were no more chances to make up with lost friends, no more chances to fix mistakes, and lastly no more childhood. I had lost the last memorable events that make up being a child and would help me transition to adulthood. College was upon me and there was nothing that could be done. It was a blow right to my soul, one that I have not recovered from yet. Losing those precious moments and that childhood security is something I was not ready for and have not fully accepted though I am working through it.

On the positive side of this situation, COVID-19 has provided me and my family with positive opportunities and has pushed us to make decisions that would have been difficult to make in normal times but became obvious decisions to us because of the pandemic. The number one thing that the pandemic has driven me and my family to do is to move upstate. COVID-19 didn't leave us a choice because the city was a breeding ground for the virus, so the obvious decision was to move. Living in a small apartment, me, my brother, and my mother had been wanting to get away from the city for many years but had never been able to due to the many ties we had with the city. Our friends were there, our schools were there, and most importantly my mother's job was located there. COVID-19 changed these things and caused school to switch to online learning, friendships to be lost, and my mother's job to no longer provide income. We are thankful for this opportunity because had this not happened, we would still be living in the city and still be complacent with our previous lifestyle. Because of the move to upstate New York our habits and routines have changed for the better. I am now able to exercise more frequently and work on losing weight while my brother is able to go on walks with me that he never took while in the city. In addition, we now have more room than in our apartment and are much more comfortable in our new house than we ever were in the apartment. Also, I have been able to see my uncle, aunt, and my cousins every day because we now live very close to them, after quarantining for a week that is.

There are many things that I will miss from the city and will not be able to experience, at least until the virus vaccine is perfected. One thing I loved about Bayside, New York was my boxing gym. Going to the boxing gym and helping out my coach and also taking boxing lessons was a crucial part of my life and had provided me with purpose. I had a duty to pass my self-defense skills on to others and was able to accomplish this through my coach and his gym. Now that the pandemic has forced my family to move, I am unable to do that anymore and in turn have lost the purpose that boxing contributed to my life. This change is not permanent because eventually the pandemic will settle down and life will return to normal and when that happens so will my return to boxing. Another thing I loved about Bayside was my school. School also provided a purpose for me and set a routine for me to follow. Waking up, getting ready for school, and doing well at school was a daily routine that became a part of me after following it for the past 18 years of my life. COVID-19 changed that and took away this routine which, I admit, was difficult at first but eventually allowed me to build a new routine, one that I have been following for the past 6 months. This routine includes exercising and interacting with my family, two things that I did not make a priority before the virus but have now become a daily blessing. Although I miss my boxing gym, my school, the great food, and many other things in Bayside I have come to terms with these losses and have been able to create something new in the devastation like a rainbow after a storm.

The previous paragraphs covered the spring of 2020, which were about adjustment and dealing with the effects of the pandemic. The summer of 2020 has been about making the best of the situation and working on improving our lives every spare moment. I have noticed many things during the pandemic and the thing that stuck out the most to me was the sense of community that the pandemic evoked. Many people made signs thanking our essential workers for continuing to help the community even at the risk of their health. People in Italy and Spain went out on their balconies and clapped and rang bells at the same time for nights in a row. This sense of community has been very powerful and has also led to people wearing masks and social distancing to protect one another. Although the pandemic has harmed many people it has also shown that people can come together and persevere through hard times, which is exactly what happened during 9/11. As the number of cases has reduced in previously hard-hit states such as New York, the world is slowly recovering from the devastation that the pandemic has caused. It is my firm belief that we as human beings are a resilient species because of our ability to recover from the hardest of times, to get up, brush off the dust and dirt, and try again. Like a forest after a natural wildfire, we come back much stronger and more experienced than before, ready to start anew as we each strive to live our lives to the fullest.

Hot Zone

August 30, 2020

ROGER W. HECHT

August is closing down, which makes it feel as if the summer is closing down, though we still officially have three weeks left till the equinox makes it official. All the late-summer flowers are out: blue cornflower, orange jewelweed, Queen Anne's lace, and a slew of others I don't know the names of. Some are already wilting. Today's cool breeze is enough to signal what's ahead in the weather. Summer's closing down. Oh, yeah, and the school is closing down. In the past five days we've gone from zero to 105 positive COVID cases, some of which must have first been symptomatic before they were reported. Someone on Facebook mapped it on a graph—the sharp upward slope of it looked impressive but it didn't look good. If only my retirement moved like that!

I expect in the coming weeks some kind of inquiry will draw conclusions about where to lay blame. To be kind, we'll say many missteps were made, such as the decision not to actually test students before they arrived on campus but to rely on self-reporting, or to not ban Greek rush **before** the parties started, or what appears to be a major lack of coordination between administration and local government and health officials—seems like much of the discussion is coming after the numbers started to climb. My information comes from conversations on many different platforms. To be kind, let's say many on campus are not pleased with the current situation.

Today the SUNY Chancellor posed an intervention and ordered what they're calling a COVID Swat Team to campus to conduct massive testing of students (and I hope staff and faculty, as well). It sounds dramatic, though I don't think it will entail either Dustin Hoffman and Morgan Freeman in Hazmat suits (though that would be impressive) or Homeland Security pulling students into unmarked vans (that would be terrifying). Still, while no one wanted this outcome, it was easy to see it coming. Why, oh why, we are asking, was this not entirely anticipated?

Part III

Fall 2020

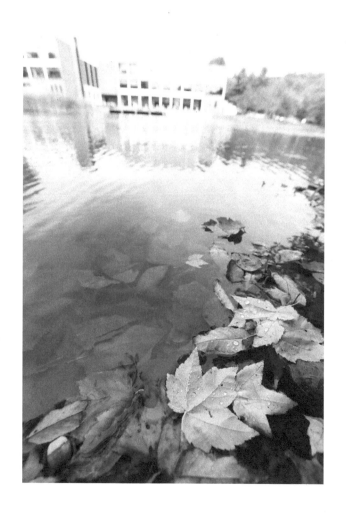

September 2020

SUNY ONEONTA

August 28–October 9—There are now 712 cumulative positives for SUNY Oneonta students.

September 3—All SUNY Oneonta classes transition to remote instruction for the rest of semester. All residential students are sent home.

September 4—Students are shown partying in Quarantine Hall on Instagram (*Barstool Oneonta*).

September 6—Students are criticized for violating safety protocols by SUNY Oneonta President Barbara Jean Morris, who announces monitoring of residence halls.

ONEONTA

September 8—Remote instruction begins at Oneonta City Schools.

NEW YORK

September 21—Pre-K and advanced special needs classes start in-person learning in NYC.

September 27—Union of NYC principals and school administrators vote "nonconfidence."

September 29—Elementary students return to public school classrooms in NYC.

USA

September 14—Pfizer, BioNTech expands phase 3 trial.

September 16—Trump administration releases vaccine distribution plan.

September 21—Johnson & Johnson begins phase 3 vaccine trial.

WORLD

September 28—Global COVID-19 deaths surpass 1 million.

Headed Home

September 3, 2020

MAKAYLA ZAMBRANO

Today I came home from college at SUNY Oneonta because of a huge COVID outbreak. I am extremely sad to leave my roommate and the friends I have made so far. I have already been robbed of so much during my senior year in high school and now it seems to have taken my freshman year of college too. I have been looking forward to this part of my life for so long. It is so hard to see it start to slip away. However, I know everyone is being affected by this virus in some way or another. I can only hope things get better in the near future. One positive thing is that now that I'm back home I will be able to focus on my academics more.

Bye, for now

September 3, 2020

Kevin Davidson

the students are
leaving now.
to homes where they
can never,
ever
concentrate.
homes where
their grandmother died.
they were abused.
they starved.
they punched holes
in the walls
and rattled
the ceiling beams
and the ceiling beams
are still shaking.
college is a chance
to reinvent yourself.
that's the line
that brought me here.
a pandemic is
a time when

inventions fail.
hordes of automatons
fighting molecules
tinier than
blood cells.
the virus wins.
the virus
always
wins.

COVID Experience Journal

September 6, 2020

Jaclyn Kennedy

9/6/20

It's Sunday, September 6th. I have been trying to be fairly careful under the new COVID-19 rules and regulations. However, I have not been staying home completely. Some friends and I went out to dinner last Friday night, September 4th. Now my group of friends that I was with is concerned we were exposed to the virus when we were out to eat. Personally, at this moment I think they are being paranoid, and I do not believe we were exposed. However, they plan to get tested tomorrow.

9/7/20

Today, my friends got tested for COVID-19. To my surprise, 4/8 of them came back positive; this included my roommate. Now of course I realize they are not paranoid, and they were more on track than I had predicted. However, it's odd . . . we were all together and yet only some of the group tested positive for the virus. Yet, since we were all potentially exposed, we must quarantine to make sure symptoms of the virus do not develop later on.

My friends who tested positive also had to share their track of who they had been in contact with. This means I was now getting calls from contact tracers. The contact tracers' job is to call people who were potentially exposed to hopefully stop the chain of exposure. Now I have found myself in quarantine . . . with my infected roommate.

9/8/20

I still have had no symptoms of the virus. My roommate and I have been extremely careful to wipe down doorknobs, clean the bathroom and kitchen (which we share), and mainly stay quarantined in our rooms so she does not infect me. At this point, I am questioning . . . How did I not get the virus? Yet, I am not the only one. My four other friends who were just as equally exposed did not get it either. With the virus being so new, I guess no one has answers as to why some are more susceptible than others at this point.

I made myself a nice dinner tonight, did laundry, did homework, and felt fine. Just as the day crept into the evening, I began to experience muscle aches (a symptom of COVID-19). I am not totally concerned at this point. Muscle aches can have a lot of causes including pulling a muscle, or simply even sleeping in a funny position. The muscle aches were not terrible, and even ignorable at this point. However, I began to be a bit concerned considering my surroundings and friends' experiences around me.

9/9/20

I slept. And slept . . . And slept some more. Something wasn't right. I finally pulled myself out of bed for the first time that day at 6:30pm, just to use the bathroom and put some food in my stomach. By 7:00pm, I was exhausted from that little bit of activity and back in bed for the night. I had come to the realization at this point, it was time to schedule a COVID-19 test. My test was scheduled for the following day, but I had a pretty good hunch of how it was going to go. The craziest part of this virus and the way it affected me personally was how quickly the symptoms crept on me. Out of nowhere almost! Just when I thought I was safe.

9/10/20

The following day was similar to the day before, I was still very very fatigued. However, today I had to force myself out of bed in order to get my COVID-19 test. Sure enough, as expected, the test came back positive. Now knowing I was positive for COVID-19, my fatigue and muscle ache symptoms made sense. However, I had already been quarantined since the past Sunday, September 6th, since my roommate and friends were infected, potentially exposing me. When I got back to my apartment, my roommate and I stopped our isolation towards each other since we were both positive at this point and began congregating in our common area together again. However, of course we still could not leave our apartment.

9/11/20

By this point, I actually woke up feeling a lot better today. I still had muscle aches, and my headaches were horrible. However, my extreme fatigue was lessening which made a big difference. I was still able to keep up with my schoolwork considering it was all online, which was good. Yet, as expected it just wasn't the first thing on my mind while being so sick. I wouldn't say I fell too behind in my schoolwork because I knew that wasn't an option for me. However, I do think my symptoms, especially the migraine, made it very hard to focus on a computer all day. I had felt like I got beat up by this virus.

9/12/20

The only positive I would say is that at least my roommate and I had each other. I was miserable enough in complete quarantine for 14 days, and I wasn't even alone. I feel very bad for people who were isolated by themselves. Once my roommate's and my symptoms began to lesson, we still had to properly finish out our quarantine, so we did not potentially infect anyone else. We spent our time in quarantine ordering a lot of delivered food and spending a lot of time on our couch. It got BORING, quick. We watched a lot of movies, caught up on schoolwork, and that's about it; but at least we had each other.

Isolating at home

September 7, 2020

MAKAYLA ZAMBRANO

Since I've gotten home, I have been isolating in my basement because I'm pretty sure I have COVID. This is scary because I live with my grandparents and my mom is prone to getting Pneumonia, so I really don't want to give it to any of them. I got tested at school and it came back negative but I'm sure that's almost impossible because my roommate and most of my friends tested positive. So far, my symptoms are minor, just achy and feel like I have a minor cold. I haven't had a fever at all this whole time, which is good, and I count myself lucky. However, when I got home, I got retested because I knew the school test was wrong: turns out I'm right and I do have COVID. They say I'm through the worst of it which is great, and I won't be contagious for much longer. It's crazy to see all these people dying from this disease and then when I get it it just feels like a little cold.

Mi horario en tiempos de pandemia

September 15, 2020

Maria Cristina Montoya

Siempre, antes y ahora, me despierto a las cuatro de la madrugada.
My Schedule in Pandemic Times

> Módulo 3 OER Español 1 y 2 "Chévere"
> Tomo seis tazas de café para despertarme.
> Saco a caminar el perro.
> Trabajo mañanas extendidas.
> Mi familia y yo pasamos todo el día en casa.
> Estamos cambiando.

> Module 3 OER Spanish 1 and 2 "Cool"
> My schedule in pandemic times
> Always, before, and now, begins at the four-dawn hour.
> I drink six cups of coffee to wake up.
> I walk the dog.
> I work extended mornings.

We are changing. My students have become pretty pictures or two letters on a screen monitor, maybe I should start calling them "Eme—Erre" "Te—Ele" and they will remember the Spanish alphabet. One month into a happy first day semester fall 2020. A world burning outside, unbalance inside, surviving and staying sane.

It shall pass, and we'll understand.
Life keeps happening . . . mi primer girasol en la vida.

Going Home

September 18, 2020

Madison Palamara

I had always been very excited to go to college. Since I can remember I would always watch YouTube videos about college so when it was my time to go, I was over the moon. I started getting ready to go to college about 2 months in advance because I just could not wait any longer. I was so excited to finally have freedom and be on my own without having anyone to check up on me. Once I got to Oneonta I knew I was going to have the best time. Within the first day I had already met so many amazing people and I was super excited to hang out with them more. We all clicked really fast, and it felt like we had all known each other for forever. Everything was going good up until the cases started to rise. At first, I wasn't nervous because this was inevitable, and all of the cases seemed to be from people off campus. Then the number kept on rising and rising and soon enough one of my friends had gotten the virus and decided to go home. After that more and more of my friends decided to go home. I was upset but I knew they had to and I thought that they would be back after they were better.

Then we got shut down by the government. I just remember how shocked everyone was and how fast this was all unfolding, but we tried to make the best of it. After a few days of this we found out we were going to be tested. I was happy that this was happening since it didn't happen before we got onto campus. Going into the testing center I was upset to say the least. To see everyone crowded in that one hall with no social distancing markers just made me angry and ultimately people could have gotten sick from just standing in that building. Soon enough it was over, and I was on our way back to my dorm with the impression I would receive my results in a matter of 2–3 days. That unfortunately did not happen, and I ended up getting my results back in 5 days. Luckily, I was negative and so was my roommate, so we weren't as worried anymore.

After about 10 minutes of receiving my results, I got the email that said we were being sent home. I could not believe my eyes and after everything that we had gone through it was over just like that. It felt like the day I found out my high school would be closed for the rest of the year and every emotion I felt then came back now. My roommate and I tried to make the best out of it the final nights we were at Oneonta. We ordered Tinos, hung out with our friends in our dorm, and had a movie night. And just like that it was time to go home. It really does suck being home but my friends and I have already set multiple dates so we can go see each other. I hope we will be back in the spring so we can finish what we have started.

Four days with a friend

September 28, 2020

Makayla Zambrano

Today is one of the happiest days I've had since I've been home. My mom drove me down to Long Island, from Westchester, and I got to stay with my roommate. I'm staying with her for four days. It's been so hard for both of us lately because our friends at home aren't the best and we just really miss school and each other. It's nice to be with her again because it reminds me of school and how we would do classes in our dorm room. This is such a lonely time for everyone, but this visit has helped so much.

Diary Entry

September 30, 2020

Tatyanna West

Diary Entry 1

Hi, I am not the best at writing diary entries because I never really know where to start. Do I start by telling you how my day had gone or by detailing my every minute. I would get so overwhelmed just trying to find a good greeting. So, I hope that you don't mind reading some of the poems that I've written over my time in quarantine. This poem is called Midnight Drum,

Heads fall nights call
Stars twinkle while eyes wrinkle
Full moon sleep soon
Beds filled and time is stilled
Finished is the daytime hum
As nighttime plays the midnight drum
Stores are closed while the stray runs through the empty rows
Low music from the park benches plays as the shadow of
    night has come to
Stay
Gentle whispers in the air telling its secret to those who'll hear
The soft cries of the motherless animal are almost inaudible
    over the roar of
the drunkard calling out for things intangible

As night continues the tasks for tomorrow are being issued
Slowly the light begins to peak past the clouds
Signaling to the night that it was time for a new sound
Alarm clocks ring TVs on
It's a new day life must go on

Diary Entry 2

Hello!! I hope you're having a great day. Today's a pretty nice day in
the city. I'm taking my nephew to the park so he can get some air after
being stuck in the house for months (not that this is his first time out of
the house lol). I made a huge mess in the kitchen last night making pizza
from scratch. Here's a poem:

Midnight Meditations

Meditative thoughts caress the soul at midnight
Looking out across the horizon
Wondering what was and will be
Polaris shines brightly over the alley
Thoughts of tomorrow weighing heavily on my mind
Stretching out longer than the cat can count
The mystery of that house down the road
Grinds the gears of your mind like the wheels of the bike you
    had at twelve
As night hides behind the coming light
Your mind begins to rest
Soft clouds take over the sky
Until tonight our song is spent

September Diary Entries

September 30, 2020

Ashley Cruz

Diary Entry 1. For me, the coronavirus greatly affected my college experience because the outbreak happened during my first semester on campus. At first, I underestimated the danger and potential, jokingly comparing it to the bubonic plague, but not really thinking it would spread out of control. I even already had plans set to go to a party after spring break ended, but unfortunately, campus closed over the course of spring break. Once the virus broke out in the US, it reached such an effect that entire spaces in New York City were deserted, which was baffling to me, as I never imagined such places could ever be empty. Even places like Times Square were empty, which really drew attention to the severity of the outbreak. During the outbreak, I also happened to be in the process of moving houses which caused lots of stress for my mom and I, as we had to move out of my old house by a certain date and I was worried I wouldn't be able to find a new house to move into in time due to the virus still putting everyone into an initial panic state. Additionally, everything was shutting down and, in the city, there was a curfew, and we weren't supposed to leave the house except to buy necessities which put more pressure on my mom and I to move quickly. As everything in New York shut down, so too did the state borders for a time, which affected me because the person who was supposed to drive me to campus to collect my things after the campus closed was across state borders and I wasn't able to get my things until May, a whole two months later.

∽

Diary Entry 2. Before the campus closed, classes were originally delayed. I had bought a bus ticket back to Oneonta and rescheduled it to accommodate for the delay, but shortly afterwards the campus and many city services closed, and I was unable to then get a refund for my now useless ticket. During the pandemic, online classes were a stressful and difficult transition. As a result of my things being stuck on campus since I couldn't get a ride back, I didn't have a computer and had to resort to buying a new one in order to do online classes at all. In terms of day-to-day living in the city, businesses had limited occupancy and long lines at best and at worst were completely shut down (which happened to many). Among the shutdown businesses were malls, where I did lots of shopping normally but couldn't go to until state borders reopened which allowed me to go into New Jersey malls since the ones in New York City were still closed. In addition to daily life disruption, many people lost their lives. Some people I knew passed away too, unfortunately, including my mom's boss, the lady who my mom took dry cleaning to, my uncle's best friend, and even a lady who baked a cake for me in day care and her husband died. In the city, the crime rate also increased during the pandemic as many people lost their jobs and faced economic hardship.

∽

Diary Entry 3. Over the summer of the pandemic, things did not go as I had originally planned. I had wanted to do veterinary work to get experience and improve my resume for entering vet school. However, because of the virus, nobody was accepting volunteers and I was stuck doing basically nothing. Most recently, I had applied to volunteer at a local shelter back at Oneonta which I wanted to work at once I returned to campus for the fall. I wound up not working there though, as I felt concerns about the stability of my return to campus. This concern proved to be accurate as shortly after returning to campus, coronavirus cases broke out and the campus sent most of its student's home. The remaining students, including myself, were kept in a two week on-campus lockdown. After the two weeks passed and the campus reopened, I didn't reapply to the shelter, as I still held concerns about the campus maybe not reopening again in the spring and I didn't want to work at the shelter for only a month or two before quitting on them and not returning. When the campus lockdown was put in place, campus dining halls closed down, which put lots of stress on the staff who suddenly had to figure a way to still feed the remaining students and for the first day there were no vegan or vegetarian options. This meant that I, a vegan, had to order from outside the campus so I would be able to eat that day. The lockdown also affected me because I had a dentist appointment for my braces, I needed to go to but I had to reschedule because of the lockdown. Additionally, after the lockdown was lifted, I encountered a second issue since I had to once again return home since my braces broke and while I was home getting them fixed, the campus informed me they were going to move me into a different dorm hall to save on maintenance costs. I was worried that I wouldn't get back in time to move out, but thankfully I was able to get back in time.

September 2020

September 30, 2020

JACOB BRESOWSKY

Diary Entry #1. The start of quarantine was not too bad for me, it was the end of high school, so I did not have that much work to do, and I started to work out again and I was feeling good. This was going on for a few months and then the summer started and I able to hang out with some of my friends again since quarantine was lifted. Then in August, I started to get breathing problems. I used to have them at the beginning of the year, but they sort of went away but in August it got worse. It would usually come out of nowhere, sometimes I would be sitting on the couch and my chest would get tight and I had to start breathing from my mouth with deep breaths. This concerned me and I told my parents about it, so we made an appointment with the cardiologist and the pulmonologist. At the cardiologist everything was fine, at the pulmonologist, I took a breathing test and the doctor said that my lungs looked enflamed and said that he would say that I am fine if I was not having trouble breathing. Since I was having trouble breathing the doctor gave me Arnuity which is supposed to help my breathing and gave me an asthma pump just in case. Since then, I have gone to the doctor one more time for a follow-up and I am going again in October. The doctor thinks it could be a mix of allergies and anxiety which would make sense because I am allergic to dust and pollen. I have had anxiety for a few years, and I guess the pandemic made it worse without me realizing it and it has not been great. The medicine has helped though so hopefully I will find out what is wrong with me soon.

∾

Diary Entry #2. Before the pandemic I was constantly active in high school. I played football for four years and lacrosse for three, so I was in pretty good shape since I was doing some type of physical activity every day for four years. Once the pandemic started, I still worked out every night and went on bike rides two to three times a week. However, once my breathing problems began, I was afraid to work out because I did not know what was wrong with me. So, I did not work out every night for a long time. Then once college started, I really did not work out anymore because I had no time to ride my bike during the day and I was too tired to work out at night. Even though I stopped working out I ate like I usually did when I would work out all the time. It never occurred to me that I did not gain weight from eating so much because I was active and when I realized that it was too late. I went from 185 pounds to 200 and now I am about 198. When I realized that I had gained this much weight I stopped eating after dinner so I would not gain any more weight. I try to work out again every once and a while, but I do not work out as much as I should because I lack motivation because I am too tired. If I were at Oneonta in normal times, I would try to go to the gym every day with my friend. When we can go to school, I hope the gym will be open so I can work out for the first time in a while. Until then who knows when I will work out again because I sure don't.

Diary Entries

September 30, 2020

ASHLEY RUSHFORD

Diary Entry #1. The year 2020 has not been for one second what I expected. It was supposed to be a great thing, something I had anticipated for most of my life, but it turned into a great mess. I am a part of the class of 2020.

Senior year is the best year of all, or at least that's what they tell you, but rather than going to prom and walking across the stage at graduation in front of my family and friends I had to sit in my bedroom and do school through a screen. Sure, it may not seem like that big of a deal, because most kids go through their school day wishing for it to be over, but once it actually is you realize just how much you miss it, because if I would've known that March 13th was the last day I would ever go to high school I probably would've cherished it a lot more. This whole experience has made me think about how much we take for granted, like going to concerts or even simple stuff like hanging out with friends. It's hard to imagine a world without those things until all of a sudden, they go away. Now we're all just waiting. No one knows what to expect in life, but I think right now the whole world is on the same page which is we have no clue what will happen next. All we can do is hope that everyone cares about getting back to "normal" life enough that they'll make the necessary sacrifices in order to have this virus end as quickly as possible.

Diary Entry #2. Quarantine is the kind of thing you hear in movies and tv shows about the apocalypse, but never expect to see firsthand. That's kind of what this whole experience has felt like, a horrible movie that doesn't seem to have an end in sight. It is the most peculiar thing when you're walking around a store, and you see that everyone is wearing a mask. It really makes you think how did this become our new normal? It seems so foreign, but at the same time it would feel just as weird to see people not distancing or wearing masks. It is something that I've struggled to get accustomed to as I'm sure everyone else is as well, but it is slowly becoming less scary. I currently have a collection of different masks all with different designs on them, and that is weirdly enough something I've enjoyed about this experience. I try to look at it as just another accessory or part of my outfit and that has definitely made it more fun. It has become hard to imagine things going back to the way they were, and I'm sure even if they do it won't be for a while. Right now, I'm attending a college that is hours away from where I'm writing this and I'm not sure when I'll be able to actually go to school. I'm hoping that I am able to experience college at some point, but for now I am just going to continue working as hard as possible while at home in order to ensure that when we all get to go back to life, I am ready.

Diary Entry #3. Music is how I have gotten through this pandemic. It is the one thing that I can always count on. I am writing this as I've just found out my favorite artist is coming out with another album and that has made me realize just how important music is to me. Music has many different emotions and without fail helps me when I am feeling anything whether it's good or bad. It allows you to travel into another world and all of the struggles you face just melt away. This pandemic has been filled with stress and chaos, but music has helped all of that get just a little bit better. It is something that is hard to put into words but listening to music is probably the most freeing thing you can experience. For that moment you are able to just live and listen, and it is almost like the artist is speaking just to you. With all of the craziness going on in the world and how unexpected everything is it is so important to be able to just relax and calm down, which is something I couldn't have done without music. I am so grateful that I live in a time where I have access to my music whenever and wherever I want, and I know that without it this pandemic would've been even harder to get through.

8

October 2020

SUNY ONEONTA

October 10–November 6—Seventeen positive cases at SUNY Oneonta.

October 15—Barbara Morris resigns as SUNY Oneonta president after 700 students tested positive, and Dennis Craig from SUNY Purchase appointed as acting president.

October 19—First day on the job for Acting President Dennis Craig.

ONEONTA

October 6—City of Oneonta Common Council mandates social distancing requirements within city limits and mask wearing when social distancing is not possible,

October 20—City of Oneonta mayor Gary Herzig vetoes Common Council social distancing and mask mandate, feeling it was unenforceable. He asks for new more narrowly focused mandate.

NEW YORK

October 1—NYC middle and high schools start in-person learning.

October 5—Governor Cuomo announces schools in NYC neighborhoods with high positivity rates must close starting October 6.

October 7—Governor Cuomo sets up red zones in New York City areas with rising COVID cases in which nonessential businesses must close, size of religious gatherings are limited to ten people, and restaurants are forced to go to take-out service only.

October 28—New York State tops 500,000 COVID cases.

USA

October 2—President Trump and First Lady test positive for COVID-19; President Trump enters Walter Reed Medical Center.

October 5—President Trump leaves hospital, continues receiving treatment. President Trump is treated with Regeneron's investigational antibody cocktail, Remdesivir, and dexamethasone.

WORLD

October 19—Global COVID cases top 40 million.

October 2020

October 3, 2020

CHELSEA SOOKRA

October 3rd, 2020. I went pumpkin picking for the first time. My sister, her best friend, my best friend, and I sped off to Long Island to pick pumpkins. Once we arrived, we were surprised by the number of people there but luckily, we were able to keep our distance.

Everyone had on their masks as well.

As we were looking to find where to pick pumpkins, we found some really nice eggplants which we had to bring home with us. After that, we found the pumpkins. We decided on the number of various sizes we were going to get and took some Instagram worthy photos. I bought some apple butter and triple crown for my mother and my sister's best friend bought apple cider donuts which were probably the best donuts we ever tasted. We went to a diner after that for lunch where the food was superb and decided to go home and call it a day.

❧

October 10th, 2020. Tonight, was my family friend's movie night. I had my reservations about going at first but once I got there, I was happy to see only a few people. The decorations really imitated a movie theater with concession stands and blankets on top of the couches. There were actually movie theater popcorn containers and little car holders to put them in. The movie DOPE was really good as well. It was my first time going out where

227

I expected there to be a lot of people despite corona but I'm glad I didn't let my worries get the best of me.

∽

October 19th, 2020. My psychology class really makes online school feel less lonesome. Despite none of us turning on our cameras, it still feels like I'm in an in-person class with them. We were able to talk about how we've been feeling because of coronavirus and that essentially every day feels like the same. Our professor shared his feelings as well and it was nice to know that he was feeling the same way we are. In fact, he almost decided to go asynchronous because what is class if he can't engage with his students. He was hopeful in regard to the new president though. He believes that we'll be able to be in person next semester and I hope so too. Sitting at my laptop in my living room all day is getting to be draining.

Fire and Ice

October 15, 2020

Ed Beck

In Rochester, NY a Zamboni caught on fire. Someone aptly pointed out that it was a nice metaphor for 2020, an ice machine that is burning. One of my friends was there for their kid's ice hockey practice, and they said the driver stayed in the driver's seat and drove the thing back to the bay where they were able to put out the fire.

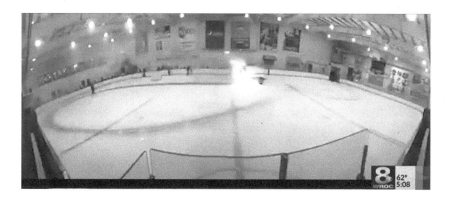

Dude literally drove a Zamboni on fire to safety. I think it's a feeling that everyone has right now. Working with instructors at my college, I just hear so much about complaints and how people aren't doing enough. Everyone is pointing fingers. Students aren't doing enough work; faculty aren't doing enough to engage with students . . . Meanwhile, every single person feels like that Zamboni driver trying to survive this year.

We all need to cut each other a little slack—students, faculty, and administration.

Deserted

October 29, 2020

MICHELLE HENDLEY

Instead of bustling with students, faculty, staff, and visitors, the campus was deserted on this beautiful fall day. Empty sidewalks. Vacant parking lots. Shuttered buildings. The long walk I took that day was simultaneously invigorating because of the sunshine and warmth and devastating because of the emptiness and silence.

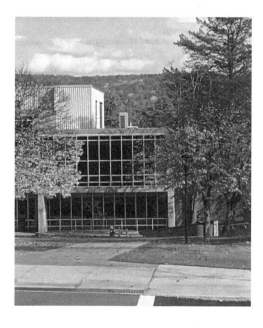

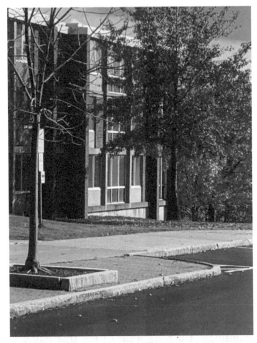

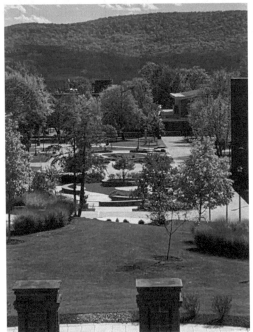

Being Positive

October 25, 2020

Makayla Zambrano

Today was a good yet simple day. I am only trying to write in this "diary" on good days because I don't want to be too negative. One of the best positives of being home for me is being able to see my half-sister. She is only one right now and every time I see her, because she doesn't live with me, she looks different. I was worried that she would forget about me when I went to college but I was only there for two weeks, so she didn't. Even though it was only two weeks away she was the one I missed the most. Now that I'm back I've been able to play with her and see her, after I was cleared of COVID of course. She even says my name now. This is one of the only reasons I'm happy to be home because lately it has been so hard for me to concentrate in school. Sitting at a computer all day just doesn't motivate me. Most days I feel tired and have a headache by the end of my lectures. I'm just hoping that Oneonta will come up with a good plan for next semester because every other SUNY school has managed to be okay so far except for us so obviously it is possible to have on-campus classes.

Diary Entries

October 30, 2020

ASHLEY RUSHFORD

Diary Entry #4

The whole situation with the virus has been strange, but something even stranger has been being a college student during it. I am currently a student at SUNY Oneonta and I am fully online. Before each of my classes I just need to roll over in bed and have virtually no prep, whereas if I was in person, I'd have to get up with enough time to make myself presentable and get to class on time. It's a weird feeling knowing you're in college, but not actually being in college. Especially since I am a freshman, I haven't experienced what college is actually like, so whenever I get to go in person it's going to be a whole new and frightening experience. Even though it's nice to not have to worry about how I look, because my camera can be off in my classes, something that hasn't been great is how hard it is to make friends. In person it is difficult to make friends, because it can be nerve wracking talking to people, but take that environment and make it completely online and making friends becomes nearly impossible. I haven't had to talk to many people and that has made college so far pretty lonely, but I'm hopeful that things will get better soon.

∾

Diary Entry #5

Trying to see your friends during a pandemic is nearly impossible. March 13, 2020, was the last day that I got to hang out with all of my friends before we were locked up in our houses for months and if I would've known I think I would've cherished it a lot more. I remember it was one of my best friend's birthdays, so we decided to all go out to eat. We talked about the virus and about how school was going to close, but no one realized how serious it was yet. This was before we had to wear masks and when we could still be in large groups and it's hard to even imagine that right now. After that night, the only time I could see my friends for months was over facetime which I was grateful for, but it still wasn't the same. I missed being able to leave my house, see my friends, and just be anywhere but my bedroom. Eventually the restrictions lightened up and I was able to see them again, but it was still different than before and I'm not sure when things will go back to normal.

೧

Diary Entry #6

I remember a few months after being in quarantine me and my friend decided we were finally going to see each other in person. We both knew we were taking the necessary precautions to avoid the virus and neither of us had symptoms or knew anyone with it, so after months we actually got to hang out in person. I went over to her house, and we went into the backyard and sat at opposite ends of the table. We were six feet apart, which is something I never thought I'd have to be from my best friend, but it was so nice to actually see another person and be somewhere else other than my house. We talked about everything and anything which was kind of crazy, because it's not like we went these months without talking, we FaceTimed and texted every day, but it's different being in person and we had no shortage of things to say.

We had lunch and coffee, and I can honestly say it was the nicest day I had had in a while. I missed seeing her and even though we had to take precautions such as staying outside and staying far apart we were actually hanging out, which is something we both really missed.

Diary Entries

October 30, 2020

Jacob Bresowsky

Recently my family and I had a COVID scare. It all started when my dad went to my uncle to get shots for testosterone because his hormones are messed up because he had two brain tumors. Two day after my dad went to get his shot my uncle called him and said that he and my aunt both had COVID. As soon as we heard this, we were all nervous because if my dad got COVID it would most likely be very dangerous because his immune system is not as strong because he had two brain humors. To make matters worse I saw my dad when he got home from my uncle's house and that same day I went to my friend's and one of them had an infant little brother who was premature. So, for obvious reasons I was very nervous for my dad, and I was afraid I had passed it on to my friend and he would pass it on to his brother. When we had found out about my aunt and uncle having COVID we got tested and my friends got tested. Miraculously no one in my house or my friends had gotten it. What is even weirder is that somehow my cousins did not get COVID even though they are in the same house as my aunt and uncle. This experience just showed me how unpredictable this virus really is.

For the past four months I have been trying to get a job anywhere and everywhere except for restaurants because that is the one place I will not work at. That is because other people's food grosses me out way too much than it should, and I cannot deal with people, especially hungry people. The places that I have applied to are Bed Bath and Beyond, Target,

US Polo, Banana Republic, GAP, Old Navy, Target, and others. I have not even gotten a reply from all these places. To make matters worse two of my friends applied to Target too and they heard back the next day and Target still has not emailed me back, safe to say I did not get that job either. I got rejected for so many jobs that my dad asked me if I did the application wrong. I think the reason that I am not getting hired is because I do not really have any good hours to work because my classes are at all times of the day. Also, I would only be able to work for two or three weekdays in the afternoon or at night and the weekend. I might try to apply to more places soon but as of right now I have lost all hope.

9

November 2020

SUNY ONEONTA

October 24–December 4—Twenty-nine people test positive for COVID at SUNY Oneonta.

ONEONTA

November 3—City of Oneonta Common Council passes mask-wearing ordinances for all public areas in city's downtown.

November 6—All Section IV high school indoor track meets canceled for the 2020–21 season.

NEW YORK

November 13—Governor Cuomo issues an order for curfews on restaurants and bars to close by 10 p.m. and limits outdoor gatherings to ten people.

November 19—Public schools in New York City are closed indefinitely.

November 20—Governor Cuomo limits indoor dining to four customers at a table and religious services to 50 percent capacity for certain areas in New York City.

USA

November 3—US presidential election.

November 4—US reports unprecedented 100,000 cases in one day.

November 9—President-Elect Biden announces COVID-19 transition team.

November 18—Pfizer, BioNTech vaccine deemed to be 95 percent effective in trials, and seeks FDA approval.

November 20—CDC warns against holiday travel.

WORLD

November 23—AstraZeneca reports vaccine is 90 percent effective.

Pandemic Halloween is a Ghost Town

November 1, 2020

MELISSA F. LAVIN

There were a few trick-or-treaters on the street tonight. Their tiny feet tapped on gravel as they walked with flashlights.

They were friendly and small, but few lit driveways greeted them. They were hungry for candy and to be loved for their costumes.

In a pandemic, Halloween is by ghosts in a ghost town.

Three Little Words

November 1, 2020

ANN TRAITOR

Three Little Words

When I was a little girl, I endlessly dreamed about being The Queen. I didn't care about the jewels or the dresses or the fancy carriages. My desire stemmed from something more basic: if I was The Queen, I would have all the power! (It is quite possible I added some evil laughter at this juncture as well.) I could make my subjects—my parents and siblings—obey me and they would be punished for their transgressions! This is a pretty enticing thought when you are 7 years old, enjoying those beautiful summer evenings, and your parents make you go to bed even though it is still light outside! Truly, a criminal act if there ever was one. Or your brother eats what was undeniably YOUR cookie—unbelievable! I had read enough fairy tales to know that I, as The Queen, could put them in a tower for their crimes forever! They would be stuck there, in their high tower room, while I ate cookies late into the summer evenings and played with my friends. It seemed so satisfying.

Fast-forward, then, many years later, to a day in my high school history class. We were talking about the preamble of the Constitution and its first words, "We the People." My teacher then said, in an off-hand way, "You can see this idea even today, when the president addresses the country at the State of the Union speech and he says, 'my fellow Americans.'" For reasons which are unclear to me even now, these words really struck a chord with me. "My fellow Americans? My fellow Americans? Wait . . . no Queen with her Queenly powers?" The axis of my thinking shifted. I started seeing America differently and my place in it differently as well.

It wasn't long before I started seeing America as a place where we really were "in this thing together," a real "res publica." Americans were helping Americans everywhere and all the time! I read about the National Guard being sent to help save midwestern farmland by piling up sandbags on the banks of the flooding Mississippi! I saw the American military use its helicopters to save people from rising waters in a hurricane! I watched as ordinary Americans did acts of kindness in their communities everyday: people finding lost pets and tracking down the owner, people volunteering to drive hot food to senior citizens with Meals on Wheels, parents cleaning up a baseball field in early spring so the Little League girls and boys would have a place to play, people planting trees and flowers to beautify their neighborhood. *My fellow Americans!*

And then there were the larger news stories too: America sends soldiers abroad to help find people buried in rubble after an earthquake! America sends food aid and medical supplies overseas to help people recovering from a hurricane! There were fun stories too: the mayors of New York and Chicago betting their own city's pizza styles in a friendly gamble on sports teams, the phrase "Beat Navy!" said at any West Point Band concert, or even the great regional debate: are they "hoagies," "subs," or "foot-longs"? *My fellow Americans!*

Those three words, "my fellow Americans," became my favorite words. I loved hearing them at the beginning of the State of the Union speech. "I am part of this union, and the President is in this too, no different from me." I was really proud to say those words, to see them in action, to be a part of this larger community of people who, although different in almost every way imaginable, were all linked together as my fellow Americans. I knew it wasn't perfect. I knew there were gaps, sometimes enormous ones, in the understanding of who, exactly, "my fellow Americans" were, but I also thought that this over-arching concept of togetherness, of people united in a common purpose, would help guide the way and see us through the rough patches into a better future.

My faith in these words has been badly shaken of late. The union I see now is no union at all. Americans are calling other Americans "the enemy." Americans are killing other Americans over skin color (have we learned nothing from the 1960s?). Americans are speaking rudely and crudely to each other (would your mother be pleased at your lack of respect?). My fellow Americans?

And it got worse. I saw Americans endangering the lives of other Americans by refusing to wear masks, Americans acting selfishly and hoarding food, medical supplies, and paper goods. I watched Americans grabbing food out of the hands of other Americans at grocery stores, Americans berating cashiers (also Americans) for not bending the rules to let them buy more than their fair share of a limited good. *My fellow Americans?* I read about Americans buying up hand sanitizer at dollar stores hoping to sell it to other Americans at 35 dollars for a 4-ounce bottle. I was stunned to see Americans flouting their wealth on social media while other Americans wait in food lines. I heard about some Americans getting great health care while other Americans have none. *My fellow Americans?*

This pandemic has not brought out the best in the US or the best in us. To be fair, there are sparks from my old "fellows"—nurses who travel to a different state to help out, health care workers who work 16 hours a day right in their own hospitals, people delivering food to the housebound, neighbors calling neighbors just to check in. But they are small sparks flying from a larger, scarier fire. I miss a lot of things in this time of sheltering down: seeing my family and friends, being able to be with students in a room all together, planning for the holidays. But the thing I miss the most is the feeling of the "us" in the US. I miss our union, in all its fragility and in all its imperfections. I want my three little words back: my fellow Americans.

Diary Entries

November 3, 2020

Ashley Rushford

Diary Entry #7:

Time this year has felt really strange. It was already eight months ago that quarantine started and that is crazy to think about. Halloween has passed and soon enough it will be Thanksgiving. At first, I felt like this year would go by slow considering that we were stuck indoors for the majority of it, but honestly, I am in awe that the year is almost over. I feel like it should still be March, and it is kind of hard to wrap my head around the fact that I am in college and I graduated high school. I think this is all so difficult to take in, because all of these accomplishments and events that have been going on have been happening while I'm still at home, but it is absolutely insane to think about. I just hope that next year brings more joy and less quarantine, because I really hope that as I go on to accomplish things, I am able to share it with the people that I care about.

Diary Entry #8:

The Coronavirus has infiltrated into every part of our daily lives. Sure, it makes sense that it has considering how scary and different it has made things, but it is also crazy to see all of the different ways that we now see references to it. This pandemic has found its way into television shows, social media, and basically everything we see. If you turn on the TV, you will see news stories about it and TV shows now have their characters living through it. I have also caught myself watching old shows where people are hanging out without masks and I have to rethink and remember that things weren't always like this, they weren't even like this at the beginning of the year. Our view of the world has drastically changed due to COVID-19, and it is kind of unsettling to think about our "new normal." However, something interesting to think about when it comes to what we're all going through is that it will be highly documented for future generations to see.

∾

Diary Entry #9:
    In today's society the internet has a major place in the daily lives of mostly everybody. People will spend hours a day on a computer whether they are writing a paper or posting on social media about what they did that day, and this will have a huge impact on how this pandemic is recorded and remembered. There are some people who are recording their daily lives to share how they've kept busy and sane when the world is currently falling apart and there are others who have decided to start blogging or even just journaling. All of these things are first-hand accounts of this life changing event that we're all living through, and they will be very important for future generations that are going to just know about the pandemic through textbooks and not through actually living during it. This is something that is unprecedented, because when we were in high school, we'd learn about events like this through black-and-white pictures and books that had accounts from a few people, but soon kids will be learning with in-depth records, and from a multitude of different people who went through this in different ways.

∾

Diary Entry #10:
    It seems as though this whole virus situation was both something that has been going on forever and something new that just started. We have been wearing masks and taking these precautions for a while now and with no end in sight, it seems as though this is just what normal life has become. Of course, this will end eventually, but I'm sure I'm not the only person who would feel that it was weird walking into a store without a mask now seeing as it's been going on for months. It has been sort of

a shock to society. All of a sudden, this pandemic hit us out of nowhere, especially in the United States because of how much the president kept from us for so long, and we just had to adapt. I think it really goes to show how strong people can be when they need to be, and for the most part people are willing to work together to bring this to an end.

Diary Entries

November 2020

Patrick Jones

November 3, 2020

Dear Diary,

Today has been a very normal day, I woke up, made breakfast, worked out, logged into my classes but there is one thing in particular that I did that was very different for me to do. Today, Tuesday November 3rd, I took part for the first time and voted in the presidential election because this year I am legal to vote. I thought this day was very important because I got to participate in my government.

Sincerely, Pat Jones

November 15, 2020

Dear Diary,

Today I started my first day of work since leaving my summer lifeguarding job. At this job I work in fields on a tree farm and do whatever manual labor my boss assigns me to do. It is very hard work, but it comes with benefits during the holidays because they do Christmas trees and I'll make good tips off of that. The most frustrating thing about this job is I have to wear a mask all day which gets in the way a lot with communication, being comfortable, etc. But in the end, it's all about others' safety and my own.

Sincerely, Pat Jones

November 26, 2020

Dear Diary,

Today is Thanksgiving. It's not my all-time favorite holiday but it was sad that it was very different this year. Instead of waking up and seeing huge crowds at the Thanksgiving Day parade there was no one watching. Instead of the balloons being pulled by hundreds of people they were being pulled by utility vehicles. It's weird to see but what was more important is that my family and I got together and celebrated the real meaning of Thanksgiving. Being thankful for each other.

Sincerely, Pat Jones

Diary Entries

November 2020

CHELSEA SOOKRA

November 3, 2020

Today was Election Day. I felt extremely nervous all day. Election Day to me was a determining factor in this country's future. I wanted Biden to win for every reason: education, immigration, climate change, and especially the pandemic. If Trump won, I knew these next four years would be just as bad as the last. If Biden won, I'll have an actual chance to go up to college and have a relatively normal college experience COVID-19 free. I stayed up all night with anticipation due to the mail-in ballots and states that took forever to count. Eventually, I called it a night exhausted from worry and the scary possibility of what tomorrow would bring.

November 22, 2020

The pandemic is really starting to get to me. I can't wait until we have a vaccine and life gets back to normal. You'd think I'd be used to it by now because it's been nine months. Alas, it feels like every day is almost exactly the same. I miss how exhilarating life used to be and all the changes every day brought. Every day is just wake up, go to class, take a break, home-work, stress, eat, repeat. Staying home is what is safest for everyone and I'm happy to do so for the greater good but the fact that we still have to do this while other countries don't really sucks. I heard that the vaccine will be out in December so I'm hoping for the small chance that maybe we'll get a normal college experience next semester.

Diary Entries

November 2020

Tanha Rani

November 5, 2020

Today the weather was really nice. I went out for a walk with just a hoodie on and it was extremely refreshing. It was pretty windy, so I held my hoodie closer to my body to gain some more heat. I looked at my phone to check the time and my eyes immediately landed on the date. How was it possible that November had started already? It felt like time was moving at a pace that I couldn't keep up with, and I was terrified, but at the same time comforted because that would mean that we might all reach a state of normalcy amidst this pandemic really soon. It feels like I don't remember much about how life was before the pandemic, but at the same time, whatever it was, I want to experience it again because I'm slowly forgetting what "normal" really is.

November 15, 2020

It was hard to get out of bed today because of the freezing weather. It felt as though I had no motivation to get up, even though I had plenty of assignments to do, and quizzes to take. Maybe it was the stress, or how every single day that went by seemed to be identical to me, that made me want to stay in bed all day and do nothing. How cool would it be to just shut your brain off for however long you wanted, and then turn it on again when you were ready to face the day and all your responsibilities again? I don't know about you, but I would for sure invest in something like that because sometimes you need to take a huge breather and just not think about anything that's going on to sort just yourself out.

Unfortunately, I wasn't lucky enough to spend a Sunday in bed, so I had to get up and start the day with an omelet and a cup of coffee. A very watery cup of coffee, but coffee, nonetheless. I opened up my Twitter feed to see if there were any interesting tweets or headlines, but there were none. Immediately after, I sat down to get my work done, and was very distracted throughout the whole process because of my mom telling me repeatedly to do my chores, but I think I did a good job of getting a pretty decent amount of work done.

November 20, 2020

I had very little to do today and was in a very happy mood because of this. Finally, being able to relax for a day, I decided to continue watching a Korean drama I started a few weeks ago and was so engaged during every episode that I finished watching the first two seasons in a day! Around 8pm, I decided to go for a train ride to the city because New York City is even more beautiful during the nighttime than it is during the day, and there's less people. I usually dread going to the city because of the number of tourists always venturing the city, but after COVID, there were way little people out on the streets than normal.

The Christmas tree at Rockefeller is always pretty, and it was equally as pretty this time around. It's bittersweet that we have to experience the holidays this way, but there is always a first time for everything so why not enjoy the holidays differently? A lot of people are not looking forward to the holidays, but I am and hope to enjoy it wholeheartedly.

November 26, 2020

Happy Indigenous People's Day! I always try to encourage everyone to try and help any indigenous people in need because many of these families are still suffering from the displacement of their ancestors, and their wealth. They are not given the facilities they need in order to thrive as a community, which in turn, leads them to live in poverty with little to no guidance or help. Today, I am thankful for being able to survive through this raging pandemic. I am thankful for my family and friends. I am also thankful for the education I am able to receive that many others around the world do not have the chance to pursue. I am thankful for being able to celebrate today with a meal on the table and a roof over my head.

Although my mom dislikes anyone bothering her in the kitchen while she cooks for us, I wanted to help with the mac n' cheese so my mom didn't mind my presence as much as she usually would. I don't think I could say I did a very good job though because it was way too runny and overcooked to everyone's disappointment so that will definitely be the last time, I set foot in the kitchen to cook for my family, but it was a learning experience!

November 29, 2020

Finals are right around the corner, and I still can't seem to let go of that holiday mind-set because I am already planning gifts for Christmas and making plans for the New Year's (but keeping in mind that we are still in a pandemic of course). I need to hit pause on all of that though and focus on the last week of the semester and finals week! Although I'm excited to finish off the semester and go on break, I am also a little upset because it was my first semester of college and it seemed to end very quickly. I had fun attending lectures and getting adjusted to the college experience regardless of the fact that I started college on different terms than I expected. This year has taught me more things about myself than ever before, and it was difficult to get through, but it taught me a lot. All in all, I hope I can pull through and not slack off in order to finish off the semester strong.

Writing out my frustrations and fears, I guess

November 12, 2020

KATHRYN KALINOSKI

I have never been more frustrated in my life. This semester is really doing a huge number on me. AND I'M ONLY TAKING 2 CLASSES. It's not just school that's frustrating me; it's really everything on top of my classes: Work, home life. I thought I didn't really have a social life before the virus, but now it really is nonexistent. It doesn't help that I'm so depressed almost all of the time, and because of life, I have no actual freedom of my own. I can't go anywhere really anyway because of virus restrictions, I have no access to a car, so I can't drive myself anywhere, which really restricts me from just leaving my neighborhood, let alone leaving my house.

I'm really struggling in one of my classes because it's hard, but it shouldn't be, but it is. Like just one aspect of it really makes it all more frustrating and confusing, and I need it to actually graduate this semester, and I just want to be done with college so badly even if it ends in this really awful situation where I don't get an in-person graduation, and I haven't seen my friends in months. The last time I saw some of my friends from college other than my roommate who lives close to me before the virus was literally on my birthday when I left for spring break. Then spring break turned into quarantine lockdown and now I'm permanently home, and I will most likely not ever see or hang out with the majority of my friends ever again.

And now I feel like even if I do graduate, which God hopefully I will this time, I don't think I'll actually feel like I actually accomplished anything. I always try to stay optimistic and positive about things, I just really want everything in my life and family's life to just get better so we can move on from all the hardships and difficulties this nightmare year from hell has put us through.

Sorry, this got kind of depressing. Obviously, I'm going through a lot, and I just wanted to write everything I was feeling and put it out there. But I'm all good and I'm going to get through all of this. And honestly writing everything I was feeling (then editing and spell checking) helped a lot 😊.

Doomscrolling

November 14, 2020

Ed Beck

Doomscrolling

The act of consuming an endless procession of negative online news.

I'm told in the original Mass Observation project someone recorded the barometric pressure and weather every day. I don't check the weather anymore; it is so rare that I leave the house. But what I have checked every day is the *New York Times* tracker of new cases. Every day, ten times a day, it has become an obsession.

Currently, we are planning how to bring students safely back to campus in February. For two consecutive semesters, we have emptied campus and sent all of our students home. It is hard to imagine how returning to campus will be possible when you compare what the national picture looked like when we sent students home in the Spring or Fall semesters when we sent students home in the fall.

Today I went to Panera to pick up takeout orders. The mall parking lot was full, and people were going about their everyday lives. Although the infection today is at a similar level to March, the attitudes of everyone around is so different. There are masks hanging from rearview mirrors, hand sanitizer in the cup rests, but we go out when we need to now. We've become accustomed to a certain level of danger.

A Dark Winter Ahead

November 15, 2020

EMMA TRUMINO

The rise in coronavirus cases across the country is concerning, and with the holidays coming up, I do not expect the rate of infection to slow down. People want to gather and celebrate with their friends and family, which is understandable, after being cooped up for so long. It is worrisome though, as the virus is so contagious, and the weather is getting colder, so outside activities are becoming limited. More people are gathering in spaces that do not have the greatest ventilation. I have remained coronavirus free so far, but that is not the case for many of the people that I know and for many people not only in the United States, but around the world. Europe is seeing a second wave of the virus and is issuing lockdowns. I am afraid the U.S. will be the next to lock down since the cases are growing so fast. The plan for the spring semester is supposed to come out soon, and I am interested to see how this will play out. It is hard to predict what will happen by the spring. There is talk of a vaccine getting approved that is over 90% effective, which is great news, but I am not sure when it will be readily available for the public, as the frontline workers will be the first to receive it. I hope it is ready sooner rather than later, as this is the only way we can return to normalcy and live our lives the way we did before this pandemic.

A break from the virus

November 15, 2020

EMMA TRUMINO

As if the year 2020 was not already historically significant enough, there is more! This time, it is a positive contribution to history, though, rather than a worldwide pandemic. The first female vice president, Kamala Harris, has been elected with president elect Joe Biden! It is so amazing to finally see a woman in such a position of power in government, no matter what political side you are on. I think that this shows young girls that they can accomplish their dreams. It is important to finally see someone like them in a position of power, rather than the same older men in office all the time. There has been much division in America recently when it comes to political views, and I am really hoping that people will become more united now with this new presidency. I think moderation is what we need, and with Joe Biden being a moderate Democrat, maybe there will be some unity between the two parties. I am a firm believer that the two extremes will never reach any common ground, but with moderation on both sides, there can be some issues that they can agree on and reach compromises, creating a political climate that is more accepting with less hatred. Everyone has the right to their own opinion, and they should never feel like they cannot freely express it to others.

Thanksgiving

November 26, 2020

Makayla Zambrano

Today is Thanksgiving and not going to lie—it's super depressing. I live with my mom and grandparents, and they all have weakened immunity, so we had to stay home. Usually, we go to my uncle's, but he didn't want to risk anything, so we stayed home, and I helped my grandma cook. However, there's a lot I'm thankful for today. Everyone in my family is healthy so far and has not been horribly affected by COVID, besides me. I still haven't got my taste and smell back completely but it is slowly improving. Another weird thing about today is the annual parade in the city was canceled. So many things just aren't the same anymore and it's hard to see an ending to this virus as it's starting to get worse again. Also, I'm stuck home next semester again which has really affected me. I just wish this could all be over soon.

November 2020

November 27, 2020

Jacob Bresowsky

This week my family and I went to a drive-in movie at a BBQ restaurant near our house. The night that we went, they were showing Elf, which is one of my favorite Christmas movies, so I was excited to go. The food there was very good, and I got a chicken tender melt which I liked a lot, and the waffle fries it came with were top-notch as well. One funny thing that happened was when my mom was trying to get the food from the waiter it fell before it went through the car window, so we had to wait a while before they gave us another one, but then it came with extra fries, and all was forgiven. In order to hear the movie, we had to tune in to a certain station on the radio, which was cool because I thought it was just going to be speakers outside. When the movie started, I could not really see it because I was all the way in the back seat, but I did not really mind because I have seen it a bunch of times, so it did not really matter if I could see it or not. At the end of the movie, we got popcorn, and I got a cookie monster milkshake which is basically just a chocolate milkshake with a bunch of chocolate chips in it and was very good. The popcorn, by far, was the worst thing about the night because it was cold and came when the movie had ended. Overall, besides the popcorn and food falling on the floor, we all had a very good time.

So, this Thanksgiving was weird. We usually go to my cousin's house in Jersey and eat in their backyard, but this year we just stayed home. It was not too bad; we watched the parade, the dog show, and football—like on any regular Thanksgiving Day. My mom made all the food, and we all helped her with something, of course. The food was great, and I was full after two plates. I could have kept going, but I wanted to save some room for dessert. Dessert was very good too. We had Pillsbury chocolate chip cookies and three different pies. I am not really a pie person, but I love cookies, and that is all the dessert I need. After dessert, my sister, mom, and I were dancing around the house singing Christmas songs. My brother sang one Disney's *Frozen* song with us and then went into his room because he is no fun and my dad usually never sings with us either, but we still had a great time. During all the songs, I picked up my dog and started to dance with her for a little bit until she had enough, and I put her down, and she ran off to the couch. Overall, it was a weird Thanksgiving, but it was still an enjoyable one.

Last week of Class

November 29, 2020

Makayla Zambrano

Today is the day before the last week of classes. I wish more than anything that I could return to campus next semester but the way the college has handled this virus, I just don't see it happening. It's really unfortunate because the college is going to lose huge amounts of money for restricting the capacity of people on campus when all the other SUNY schools were able to achieve a semester without a shut down. All SUNY schools deserve to be treated the same but that is not what's happening. This virus has made me realize one thing: life is not fair at all.

Last 8 am of the Semester

November 30, 2020

MAKAYLA ZAMBRANO

Today was my last 8 am lab for this semester! I'm so happy that I won't have to wake up that early anymore, at least for a little while. However, it makes me think about how this pandemic has affected my education. Remote learning is definitely not the same experience as in person learning. I'd say that there are pros and cons to it though. For example, I can go to class in my pajamas and when I had my 8 am I only got up 5 minutes before and turned on my computer. If I was on campus, I would have had to actually get ready and walk to class. Also, a lot of tests are open book now which is great for the time being. However, I'm probably not retaining as much information as I would be if I was learning in person. I also feel like some of my professors sort of gave up with online teaching because they can't do it as effectively. Even though online learning comes with its positives, I'd give it up to be in person and receive a quality education. Hopefully, next fall will allow me to do that.

Part IV

Winter 2020–21

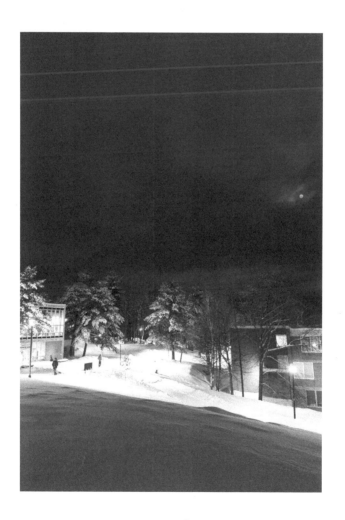

10

December 2020

SUNY ONEONTA

December 7—Last day of class at SUNY Oneonta.

ONEONTA

December 11—New York high schools cancel all winter sports.

December 23—Bassett Healthcare Network begins first COVID vaccinations of health-care workers in Otsego County.

NEW YORK

December 14—The first public doses of Pfizer, BioNTech's COVID vaccine in the US is given to health-care workers in New York City (originally made available only to people seventy-five and older, health-care workers, nursing home patients, teachers, and other vulnerable essential workers).

December 14—Governor Cuomo orders indoor dining closed in New York City.

December 21—Senator Schumer announces New York State to receive $9 billion from federal COVID relief bill.

December 30—Governor Cuomo updates quarantine requirements for exposed individuals without symptoms down to ten days from fourteen days.

USA

December 11—FDA agrees to emergency use authorization (EUA) for COVID-19 vaccine from Pfizer, BioNTech. Shipments begin to vaccination sites.

December 18—FDA signs off on EUA for Moderna's COVID-19 vaccine. Shipments begin to vaccination sites.

December 21—New COVID-19 variant circling the UK.

December 31—US falls short of goal to give 20 million vaccinations by year end. Only about 2.8 million have received their initial COVID vaccine doses.

WORLD

December 29—Eighty million cases of COVID worldwide thus far and 1.8 million deaths.

My COVID Experience: January–December 2020

December 5, 2020

CLIFFORD O. SWEEZEY

The COVID-19 pandemic will infamously be remembered at large for face masks, Zoom meetings, toilet paper shortages, and six-foot distance markers. But beyond that, the pandemic has certainly affected everyone's lives differently. My own trials and tribulations have beaten me down, yet the events of the pandemic have allowed me to adapt, grow, and learn. I'll try my best to summarize the pandemic through my own life events to offer a bit of personal history that I can look back on sometime and say, "Did all that really happen?"

It's fair to say that I think many of us were naive to think COVID-19 would never find its way to the United States. Recent studies have shown that the virus may have been here months before its outbreak, as early as December 2019, with all of us living our lives as usual. I'll never forget I went to a Team Trivia night on the Oneonta campus with a few friends, either toward the end of the Fall 2019 semester or the beginning of Spring 2020. One of the current events questions was to name the scientific name for the virus. We all knew it was the coronavirus, but we had no clue it was officially called COVID-19. Another omen came when I was home for winter break with my girlfriend, and we spent one night watching Netflix. One series we enjoy watching every now and then is *Vox: Explained*, which has truly interesting episodes on current issues. Released in November 2019 was an episode titled, "The Next Pandemic." Scientists, academics, and even Bill Gates all chimed in on why the next major world crisis would be one of public health due to several reasons such as poor preparations, overpopulation of both humans and animals, and plain inevitability.

I actually got fairly ill around the time of the Super Bowl and Iowa Caucus for reference. I woke up in the middle of the night with chills, sweats, and nausea, a sickness I had never felt before. I got up at seven in the morning and went to the Urgent Care clinic to be first in the door for an appointment as fresh snow was covering my car outside Matteson Hall. I was tested for the flu, which came back negative, and the professional that examined me claimed that I had a sinus infection and gave me some general over the counter drugs to help. I felt this way for several days, with my symptoms disappearing suddenly one day as I returned to class and other activities. Was it COVID in its infancy and I just didn't know? The answer is I'll never know for certain since COVID wasn't even a thought in anyone's mind, and all I can do is ponder the thought. I know a few family members and even friends on campus that got sick around the same time and chalked it up to being some sort of cold. But despite all of this, and as the virus did find its way onto US soil in faraway states like Washington, I still felt very safe on campus because that's the place where students had been for the last two months. I circulated the thought of students just staying on campus instead of going home for spring break in early March to try and maintain a bubble. That would not be the case as thousands of students on Oneonta's campus, and millions of other college students around the country traveled home for their own spring breaks, and that was the beginning of the end in my mind . . .

I left campus for spring break on March 6, I dropped off an assignment to Dr. Harder in her office before I departed in the morning, and even worked a few campus tours for my admissions job. With the virus slowly but also rapidly spreading throughout the state and the country, I was optimistically looking forward to my spring break. In my mind, spring break is the halfway point in the semester where I can reset, take some time off, and get ready to tackle the hardest weeks of the year. My girlfriend was celebrating her birthday on the seventh, my own birthday on the ninth, and I was able to help my old high school with its baseball tryouts for the week as I'm pursuing my career in secondary social studies education and hopefully coaching baseball as well.

But the home that I was returning to was already a broken one to begin with. In short, my parents have always had their issues with one another, making for a difficult home environment growing up and still through my college years. On top of which, one of my parents has been a hypochondriac for at least the entirety of my life, so the eminent outbreak of the virus had put them in a tailspin while I was home. Those anxieties mixed with the dysfunction with their spouse culminated into a turbulent environment to say the least. I found myself getting stuck in between arguments of my parents, over whether or not I should be working at the high school that week, or if we should even go out to dinner on my birthday. All of which rattled my head, waiting to be able to go back to my dorm and have some peace and quiet.

But for the time being, that peace and quiet, or more so a tranquility came about when I was in fact working at the school that week. Despite hearing about the spread, and the eventual shut down of the SUNY system and my extended spring break, it was great to catch up with old teachers, talk about how to go about my future to become an educator, and run tryouts for the JV baseball team that I once played for a few years prior. Baseball has always been a passion of mine, playing since I was 4 years old. It came naturally to me, and the game has offered me so many experiences and stories that I'll always be grateful for. A season-ending shoulder injury my senior year of high school ended any future playing days I had going into college, so I see it that I'm starting my coaching career ahead of schedule. If anything, coaching has helped me realize that educating, both in the classroom and on a ball field, is how I want to make an impact in this world. But after a few hours of being in my element, the talks of COVID would of course come up between my other coaches and the students. It always came up at the end of the day making sure to wash our hands and not to share anything that we normally would. High fives soon turned to fist bumps, and ironically on Friday the 13th was when everything started to go downhill . . .

It seems to be a cliche that things are always going so well before they go downhill, and this was the case. I was actually left on my own to run the practice that day as the other coaches had to attend a mandatory meeting with our athletic director to of course discuss the pandemic. In the meantime, I was left on a warm and gorgeous Friday afternoon to throw batting practice, get pitchers throwing bullpens, and keep everyone active and involved. I told the kids that today was their last day to stand out in some way, and to leave it all out on the field, and they seemed surprisingly motivated and eager to do so. But about an hour or so into practice, the other coaches came back from their meeting, and we continued as usual until our athletic director came out on his famous golf cart and stopped our practice dead in its tracks, told us we had to pack up and be off school property by 4:00 sharp. The district was shutting down for two weeks as everyone was going to stay home and see what happens with the virus. That's when it started to hit me that things are starting to get a little off the rails. But at that point, I had to act the part of my athletic director and other coaches to be reassured that everything was going to be fine in no time and that we just had to take a break for a bit. How wrong we would all be.

With the ever-increasing threat of the virus being in our community, things at my home had gotten so bad that I ended up staying at my girl-friend's house for the time being while most of her family was actually in Las Vegas on vacation. In the time being, she and I were basically keeping the house in shape and making dinner for us and her two younger broth-ers. During this time, I remember going out a few times to the stores to get groceries, and at this point in time there were no mask mandates, and neither was there any toilet paper or cleaning supplies on any shelf in any store you walked into. Regular food aisles weren't wiped clean but were definitely being bought beyond normal buying habits. People were certainly preparing for the worst, and it was an eerie feeling being in stores with no masks, everyone kind of eyeballing one another as we'd walk past as we were all in this state of limbo between life as we knew it and what was to be. In the meantime, one of my girlfriend's uncles who works in the airline industry gave word to her mother that they had to get out of Vegas as soon as possible before they shut down the airlines and they were going to be stuck there. Sure enough, they came home on one of the last flights before everything shut down. With them coming back, there wasn't any room for me to stay any longer so I tried to put up with things at home, but I just couldn't.

Just like dominoes falling, I then got word that students were not to be allowed back on campus and that I had to set up a time to move out of my room. At the time, my only hope and vision was that I could get back on campus and be away from home again and things will be back to normal. But then thoughts about how things such as dining halls and other campus resources would be maintained amidst the pandemic made me understand why campus had to be shut down, and I came to terms with that. And just like every other college student, I had the tail end of my semester to finish and knew that I simply couldn't do so at the expectations I set for myself, living in the house that I was in. Fortunately, an aunt of mine reached out to me well aware of what was going on at home and offered that I come ride this thing out with her in Groton, Massachusetts, a whole four hours away from home. I knew in the beginning that any contact with anyone during quarantine would be limited to none but going away to Massachusetts meant not seeing anyone at all aside from my aunt and her boyfriend that she lives with (who is practically an uncle to me now). It was really a tough decision to make, knowing that I wouldn't be able to spend any sort of time with my girlfriend or any other friends, but I knew what the right answer was. In my mind, I just needed somewhere to spend some time to clear my head from my mess at home and finish my semester strong.

March 20th was when I packed my few things that I had brought home for spring break and went back up to the Oneonta campus to move myself out of my room on my own. As I pulled away from my house and to then say goodbye to my girlfriend, the song *Life in a Northern Town* by The Dream Academy was the first song to play in my car. It was just one of those moments that you know you're never going to forget, especially with all of the thoughts and emotions that were running through my head at that point. I made good time driving up to Oneonta from Long Island, since many people had already started to stay home. It was mostly a cloudy drive up, and I couldn't help but notice how cheap gas had gotten in such a short amount of time as I drove through the small towns of the Catskill region. When I arrived on campus, I of course realized that it was an absolute ghost town. There was a phone number I had to call to inform residence life that I had arrived and was ready to move out. I don't think there was one other person in Matteson Hall, at least in the few hours that I was there packing my things up, and then lugging them downstairs and shoving them into any open space I could find in my car. Already exhausted, the drive up and move out was only half of my journey that day as I then had to drive another four hours east to Groton. In between, I grabbed a bite to eat at Wendy's and filled up my gas tank at Mirabito and headed off. I don't remember what time I got there exactly, but it was late at night, I was beat, and my aunt was about to go to bed after I had gotten in the door. What I find funny looking back is that I was about 10 minutes away from the house when I was stopped by a late-night freight train coming through some dark, random intersection that my GPS had led me to. I probably waited at least 15 minutes for the train to pass, and in the meantime, I gave my aunt and girlfriend a call that I had just about made it. By the time I got there, I was so tired that I just left everything in my car, went inside, said a quick hi and goodnight to my aunt and fell right asleep.

The next morning, I unpacked my car and got my spaces set up around the house. I was very fortunate that I was offered a bedroom of course, as well as a dining room that was never used to become my "office" for the time being, and a den in the basement for me to hang out in to play video games with friends, watch TV, or work out. I had finally gotten the peace and quiet that I had needed after being home, but I never thought that I would spend the next two months tucked away from society in rural Massachusetts. One of my first days there, my aunt and I went on a walk through the neighborhood that led us to a nearby dog park. Roundtrip, it was probably about an hour and change, as we discussed all sorts of pandemic related thoughts and concerns. She and I also made trips to the supermarket to get out of the house, with still no masks required out in public. After coming home, my aunt would wash all the food before putting it away, something that I'm sure none of us do as of December 2020 with case counts completely blowing out those of late-March and early-April. Some other memories that I have while in Mass would be either overhearing the news in the background as we ate dinner or watching it directly after. Much of the time was President Trump holding his daily press briefings that left many people, myself and my aunt included, baffled, and confused as the nation faced the increasing outbreak. Looking back, it is odd to realize that that period of time was really only the beginning, but having lived through it, it had felt like months at the time for some reason. Time for me was truly either altered or out of the window. By the time I had left Massachusetts, it had been two very long months in my mind. Part of that could be because I found myself in a very abnormal sleep schedule, especially for a college student, waking up no earlier than noon just about all the time, and not being able to fall asleep until after two in the morning. That can of course be chalked up to emotions, anxieties, and stress that we have all felt at some point during this pandemic.

That being said, I generally didn't have a great amount of motivation to do anything productive initially. Thankfully, the final six weeks or so of my semester weren't necessarily demanding. I had three research papers to write by semester's end for my history classes, with a few assignments scattered in for my political science and Italian classes. Seeing the rest of the semester as "just six weeks" before I could truly kick back and relax, I was able to dedicate enough hard work and efforts to earn myself a perfect 4.0 GPA for the semester, putting me on the Provost List. I spent much of my leisure time on FaceTime with my girlfriend, playing video games with friends back home, chatting with my aunt and her boyfriend, or simply spending alone time with myself. As winter slowly shifted to spring, I tried getting myself into running as a way to get out of the house and get some fresh air, but that phase was over very quickly. However, there is one beautiful spring day in particular that I remember quite well. It was probably early May, and it was a seasonably warm day, probably around 70 degrees but at this point in the year it felt like a warm summer day. There weren't any clouds in the sky, and my aunt had just bought a badminton set for the backyard. I just remember having a good time outside and, in the sun, and after an afternoon of fun with the sun setting at an appropriate time, it was like that feeling that people get as kids after they get home from a day at the beach, waiting for dinner. And I did have myself a delicious dinner prepared by my aunt: stuffed pasta shells with sausage and a nice house salad. For that day, everything felt okay in my world. Afterwards, I wasn't too sure what I had to look forward to as summer neared. I know that I wanted to see my girlfriend and friends, but how could I do so while going back to the home that I had just gotten away from, wounds still very fresh between me and my parents.

Just as those thoughts began to kick in, I had heard from another aunt of mine who lived back home on Long Island in Port Jefferson. Her and my uncle had a tenant in an apartment above their house who was leaving June 1, with neither of them willing to rent it out again because of the pandemic. I finally had something new to look forward to; summertime, being back home, and having my own "place." Towards the end of May, I began getting myself ready to return home. A roughly 45-minute drive from my hometown to see my girlfriend and friends sounded a whole lot better than four hours. I shaved my face for the first time in two months. I got my haircut just as Massachusetts had reopened barber shops and salons, and I recall having a very nice conversation through my mask with the woman that cut my hair.

I spent my first night back on Long Island with my parents so I could unload things I didn't need as well as gather other things like my summer clothes. Being tucked away for two months meant I couldn't possibly have any trace of COVID in me, so it was okay with them for me to stay the night so I could see my girlfriend the next day. The next morning, I drove to her house with a smile from ear to ear on my face, giving her a big hug and kiss as soon as I got out of my car. Despite being physically apart for so long, her calls and texts definitely helped me get through the issues that I had faced in those few months.

My summer turned out to be one of the most productive ones that I've ever had. Despite everything going on that I had mentioned, I had taken a summer class on Tsarist Russia so that I could lessen my course load for the upcoming school year. I have been a Door Dash driver for almost two years, doing it every now and then in my spare time, and did so a few times during the pandemic where I averaged making about $20/hr! I also was able to work a virtual internship with the Greater Oneonta Historical Society (GOHS), in which I helped the executive director create a webpage about the historic Damaschke Baseball Field in Oneonta. Then in about mid-June, I was contacted by the travel baseball team that I coach with asking if I wanted to coach with them in the condensed season they had for the summer. I never thought they would be able to get any sort of season put together. Either way, I took them up on it, as it really only came down to a few weeks' worth of games, practices, and tournaments that I had to work. It proved to be an enjoyable season between the kids that I was able to coach, as well as my head coach who offered me plenty of insights and tips that I'll use moving forward. I even got myself a job lined up for when I moved back up to Oneonta in August to an off-campus house with my girlfriend and a few other friends. I even began to delve into personal finances as I opened a couple credit cards for myself and started investing. Just like with my aunt in Massachusetts, spending a few months with this aunt and uncle of mine helped me build even better relationships that I have with each of them. It was a busy and enjoyable summer, despite the wider circumstances going on in the world.

I was beyond excited for the Fall 2020 semester to get started. My friends and I found a really nice house in Oneonta to call home for the year, and with all-virtual classes for me to begin with, I had my part-time job to give me some sort of commute and time out of the house each week. I felt like I had the smallest bit of normalcy back in my life. Despite the outbreak on campus, I had a pretty smooth start to the school year between classes and work. My roommate and I would spend the last month or so of the summer having a catch down at Neahwa Park, hitting the driving range, or playing some tennis on campus. Nights were hot in our house, no AC, windows open, fans blasting.

But as summer became fall, things became a bit hectic for me. School work began piling up at the same time that I had spent over $1500 on tickets to go to the World Series in Arlington, Texas in hopes that I would see my Yankees in a truly once-in-a-lifetime experience. On top of which, I had been contacted by the NYS Contact Tracing Program for a part-time job that I applied to way back in the spring. I ended up taking them up on that offer as my other job in town didn't pay nearly as much as contact tracing, and it was all at-home work with no risk of being in public with rising cases, etc. I've been working that job since October, and it has been a really great experience. As soon as I had made that decision, I realized I then couldn't risk traveling all the way to Texas for a two-day excursion, especially after the Yankees were eliminated from the playoffs. I ended up selling those tickets, making a nice profit, and was able to settle into my new job, while also being able to handle my schoolwork that was piling up on me.

I'm heading into the end of the Fall 2020 semester with high hopes. I was able to survive another semester of online learning, hopefully with another 4.0 in the mix. I also landed a substitute teaching position at my old high school for when I'm home for break and after graduation, barring that K–12 schools aren't shut down anytime soon. I currently have grad school applications to submit, and the GRE to take in January so I can move along with my studies and career ambitions of becoming a 7–12 social studies teacher. As far as my current studies, I have one semester left before I graduate. I'm enrolled in my senior research seminar for history which includes writing a 20–25-page research paper (yikes!). However, I only have three other classes to take, with no classes on Fridays so I am very much looking forward to my three-day weekends. Although the pandemic is at its worst point so far, I am surprisingly optimistic about the future as graduation is only months away, and grad school just around the corner with hopefully plenty of experiences waiting to be had as the pandemic can hopefully be tamed by then.

At this point, I'd like to thank those who were able to offer this opportunity to write about our own experiences during the pandemic. For me, this offered me a bit of therapy and reflection from the last few months, in what will go down as one of the craziest years in history and my own personal life. I hope that you can find some sort of enjoyment, enlightenment, and/or use from reading this as COVID-19 hopefully becomes a piece of the past.

My COVID year

December 12, 2020

MERTON D. SHELDON

It was a cold morning in early March of 2020. I do not normally listen to the news on the radio, but I was beginning to become concerned about this virus that seemed to be spreading worldwide, the newscaster called this virus COVID-19. As I continued to listen on my way to campus, the reality of this situation began to sink in. I thought, "This is going to become a serious problem." What I did not know then was how serious a problem it would become. As I pulled into the SUNY Oneonta commuter parking lot, just in time for my 11:30 AM history of Soviet Russia class, I shut the car off. I did not realize this would be the last time I would be on campus to attend classes.

As my day progressed, other students and I began talking about all of the sports leagues that were just put on "pause" because of the growing concern over the virus. As we spoke about the cancellations someone brought up the question if we would be able to come back to campus after spring break. I immediately said, "Of course we will come back." I never dreamed that this would become a global pandemic that has affected everyone's life in some way. At the time I simply thought that medical professionals would come up with some type of treatment before it got that bad. Boy, was I wrong on so many levels.

On my way home from campus the final day before spring break, I again listened to the news on the radio. The newscaster had a guest on her show, the guest was a professor of Infectious Diseases at some Ivy League

278

University. The doctor was telling of the precautions people could take to limit their risk of catching COVID-19. He spoke about masks and handwashing. I thought to myself, handwashing should always be a top priority, but there is no way anybody going to wear a mask in public. Once again, I could not have been more wrong. I think that like many other people I did not want to face the reality of this pandemic, so I just minimized it and hoped it would just go away. If you would have told me nine months later, I would be sitting in my living room writing this blog, still in the middle of a pandemic I would have said you are lying or simply wrong.

Over the next week the slow drip of cancellations and postponements became a tidal wave. First it was the NCAA Basketball tournaments, then professional basketball and baseball. The Olympics and tennis tournaments were cancelled next. Finally, these cancellations hit home as my daughters' school was going to be closed for two weeks. After that they would be attending virtually from home. I remember saying to my wife, "How did we get here?" Is no one who is in charge of anything in this Country or World capable of stopping this? The sad answer to my question was, of course, no. The next couple of days brought no good news on this front. Businesses would have to shut down, people were going to be out of work, making them vulnerable to food and shelter insecurities. It was becoming clearer that this was going to last a while, and people were going to suffer, and in many cases even die. As the days went on finally, we got the word that the college as well as all other SUNY schools, were going to be closed for the rest of the semester, and we would shift to an entirely online model of education.

The college cancellation came as a surprise to me, even though it should not have. Quickly the school shifted to online classes only. This was a bit of an adjustment for me. I do not do well with online classes. I would much rather be in a classroom, but sadly this was no longer an option. The slow trickle of news from the school was maddening. I do realize that the college was just trying to keep everyone informed, and that there is no precedent for our current situation. But that being said, the emails that something else on campus was cancelled or postponed that came daily the first month of the lockdown was depressing. I feel one email with all of the cancellations and postponements would have been better. I am not trying to fault anyone; this is just my opinion.

The shift to online learning went much better than I expected. All of my professors were able to adjust their method of teaching and implement the new system. This must have been a monumental task, but they all did it like professionals. The hardest part for me with online classes is simply staying on schedule. I do much better with a rigid schedule that does not allow me the opportunity to procrastinate. With the help of all of my professors, all of which were extremely understanding of any difficulties I had, I was able to overcome my character flaws and have a successful semester. The worst part of online classes became the isolation. I enjoy being on campus and around people, I love the back-and-forth discussions that are so hard to duplicate with a class that is conducted over Microsoft Teams or Blackboard. But once again, my professors would not stop at anything to replicate this as best they could, given the current circumstances.

As the spring semester drew to a close, I thought that things were starting to look up and we would be back on campus in the fall. This gave me hope that things would soon go back to some type of normalcy. I ended up taking a summer course because I discovered that online courses were not that bad, and I should not be afraid to utilize them. This went well too, again the professor was incredible, and I feel that I got every bit the education that I would have received in a classroom setting. In fact, the class I took was the history of New York City and it was one of my favorite classes to date at Oneonta. The class started with the Dutch settling the city and ended with modern times. I would highly recommend this course to anyone who has a love for history. My summer was actually pretty good considering the current situation. I am sort of a homebody, so I do not go many places anyway, so the restrictions did not have much of an effect on my day-to-day life, other than financial implications of no longer having a place to work.

On a personal note, I am a non-traditional student at SUNY Oneonta. I am a bit older than my fellow students and I am married with children. The hardest part of this pandemic for me was always being scared. Scared that my wife or kids would get sick. Scared that I would get sick and end up in the hospital all by myself. The fear was almost constant, and at points was all-consuming. My wife is an emergency room nurse, at a hospital an hour or so outside of New York City, right in the heart of the outbreak. This was extremely stressful for us as a family. My wife lived in fear that she would bring the illness home, as well as being overwhelmed by patients at work. Watching my partner in life and my best friend be burnt out by constant stress and being overworked was difficult. But like always she handled it like a champ and never wavered in her duties as a health-care professional. As I sit here writing this, we are over nine months into a pandemic that I thought would never happen. But we have hope, there are several vaccines that are set to be distributed soon. We can only hope that they work, and we can return to some form of normalcy in the future.

11

January 2021

SUNY ONEONTA

January 24—SUNY Chancellor Jim Malatras announces weekly COVID testing for all students and staff during SUNY Oneonta visit.

January 25—Classes begin in SUNY Oneonta with 80 percent remote and 20 percent dual modality.

ONEONTA

January 24—SUNY Chancellor Jim Malatras announces SUNY Oneonta is recommended to be COVID mass vaccination site.

NEW YORK

January 4—Governor Cuomo announces expanded vaccine availability to all front-line health-care workers providing in-person care.

January 12—Governor Cuomo expands phase 1b of the state's vaccination plan to include individuals aged sixty-five and older and immunocompromised individuals.

USA

January 6—Department of Health and Human Services to provide $22 billion to fund testing and vaccine distribution.

January 8—Pharmacies are allowed to distribute vaccines.

January 19—Pfizer, Moderna, AstraZeneca to test vaccines in adolescents.

WORLD

January 4—UK begins distributing AstraZeneca/Oxford vaccine.

January 5—Moderna to produce 600 million vaccine doses.

A semester during COVID

January 8, 2021

RAYMOND SCLAFANI

Editor's Note: The following entries were originally posted in January 2021, as retrospective multiday entries that reflected on the fall semester.

Diary Entry 4:

My housemates and I decided to make an agreement with one other house that we were only allowed to see each other so that we could still have that social interaction that was outside of our immediate household. This plan worked out really well since none of us ever contracted the virus and we were still able to see people; I wish other people thought of this rather than having an explosion of cases in the town. The cops really cracked down this semester, one night the four of us were sitting on our front porch just playing cards and an officer pulled up to our house and told us that they received a "noise complaint" but we were pretty sure he just saw that we had colored lights on and assumed that there was a party going on. No harm done though; he was just doing his job, which was fine.

❧

Diary Entry 5:

The four of us got tested at Urgent Care and we all tested negative of course since we were being so careful, which I was very thankful for. The school also started offering free testing for students, which I took full advantage of. I started getting tested once a week to make sure that I was always healthy since I knew that I would not be able to go home unless I was completely sure that I was negative for COVID. I am really glad the school offered these tests to us; I just wish that they would have been more careful at the beginning rather than after learning what happens when you put a few thousand kids in dorms together that haven't been outside in months the hard way. Classes have been challenging for me this semester, it makes things especially harder when professors do not respond to my emails after I follow up with them three times since there are not many other ways to contact them during this time. While I understand that they are getting swamped with emails from students and the board, if I ask you in class if you saw my email and you say "yes" after a week of no response it hurts a little to know that you just did not want to answer my questions and help me to succeed in your class.

∾

Diary Entry 6:

I finally came home after spending August-November in Oneonta for Thanksgiving. I got tested every week for the six weeks leading up to the break to make sure that I was always healthy. I was negative every time which I'm grateful for, but not really surprised. However, a few days after coming home my sister tested positive for COVID. She either got it from her boss or from her boyfriend; we still are not entirely sure. Just my luck to be so careful for months in the coronavirus central in New York state for months just to come home and get it before the holiday. Thankfully, my father never got it since we had not been to his house since my sister's exposure, so he was able to drop off any supplies that we needed. We were very lucky because my brother and my sister never actually showed any symptoms, but my mom and I did. I actually had it the worst out of everyone in my family oddly enough, I felt absolutely terrible for about five days but then it just went away, it was a very weird virus to contract. It did not last a terribly long time, but it hit hard.

∾

Diary Entry 7:

Everyone in my family successfully recovered from COVID, I am very thankful for that. I am glad that we did not add to the number of deaths in the country, we were very lucky. This semester has been one that I will never forget, it was easily the most challenging one that I have ever experienced in my 7 semesters as a college student. I learned a lot about the people close to me and where they stood on certain aspects of life, like public safety and awareness, as some just did not care and thought their rights were being restricted for some reason. The main thing I learned is that people only care about other people in the beginning of a global crisis. Once a month or two passes a lot of people just stop caring and do whatever they feel like for their own selfishness. It was quite eye opening, and I hope that the vaccine is a success for the world so we can start returning to our lives at least in some respects.

My Life Before and Now

January 8, 2021

Joseph Trombetta

I became interested in this blog because I feel as though I am ready to share my experience before and after COVID. I have undergone a period of mental growth over the last year and a half.

Before I begin my discussion of my student life during quarantine, I must provide some context of my life prior to COVID. In fall 2019, I started my time as a student at SUNY Oneonta after transferring from a private institution. I had worked hard and scored highly in my classes during my first semester at Oneonta. I even attended some club meetings in my spare time and bonded with certain professors. You might conclude I really enjoyed my first semester at Oneonta, and while I cannot say it was unenjoyable, I knew I was not feeling well at the time. Around that time, I had dealt with several recent losses in my family. In fact, my first day in Oneonta occurred after a funeral the day prior. Hence, I was very overwhelmed emotionally to say the least. So, how then did I score highly my first semester? I have since realized, with some outside assistance, that I funneled all the painful energy into my studies and used it to distract myself from emotions. Of course, I try my hardest in my classes for the simple sake of doing well academically, but that semester my studies carried undertones. The intense focus I placed on school made me very critical of myself and I felt as though I could not relax. I would put myself down and question if I had the capacity to understand my subjects, critique that I was not doing well enough even though I was, among a multitude of other negative comments. With that came doubts of my future in terms of finding a career. All this energy was only compounded by my status as a new transfer, and with that the pursuit of friends while balancing studies.

Perhaps the hardest thing that I had to deal with that semester was the feelings of isolation and loneliness. I am reserved to myself for the most part, except when I can feel a special connection with a person. When I started the semester, I was worried if this introversion would hinder me from meeting people, and to an extent it did, though I give myself credit for trying as much as I could. Nevertheless, I struggled to find my niche, and much like with the emotions of loss I had, I focused myself into my studies to distract from the feelings of loneliness. As I had stated, I did make efforts to socialize. One club that I attended during this time was the campus's NAMI—National Alliance on Mental Illness. NAMI's mission is to educate and provide supportive information for mental health related issues. At this time, I feel that it is appropriate to acknowledge that I have struggled with problems that have stemmed from my Obsessive-Compulsive Disorder (OCD). I feel this is a necessary point to add as it may provide context for why I fell into a cycle of self-criticism during my first semester. In brief, OCD has two components, the obsession and the compulsion, or action done for relief. Therefore, the obsession in the situation of my first semester was my academics and the compulsions—relief measures—included tasks such as checking my grades frequently. NAMI proved to be a beneficial outlet in helping me cope with problems such as these during this time. However, I continued to struggle mentally, though my path toward mental liberation was just beginning.

As spring 2020 began, I was feeling somewhat better, though there was area for improvement. This semester was the beginning of my mental growth. Over the course of the semester I received various treatments, which helped me comprehend why I was self-critical and how to alter my thought process. I likewise started to realize at this time how emotional pain such as familial loss can contribute to the mind-set I had in the fall. I was able to feel less introverted and started to make friends through organizations such as NAMI as a member of the E-Board. I also joined the Oneonta State Emergency Squad (OSES) as a probationary student. I was taking a lot more initiative to feel better. I especially learned the importance of balancing school and social activity that semester, and I am continuing to learn how to do so. I started off well in all my classes, though as the semester progressed, I struggled in one of them. Nevertheless, things began to set in to place and I felt more connected to the campus community. I was beginning to feel well about myself. I engaged in old hobbies, such as model building, that I had once given up. However, as we all know, this was the semester when learning transitioned to online and campus extracurriculars ended. While there is never a good time for a pandemic, I thought the timing was very poor in terms of the progress I was making. After some self-reflection, I did not let the transition to online get me down, though like most I was initially disgruntled with the change. Despite this hinderance, I finished out the semester as best I could on the new platform.

Fall 2020, the semester that could have been. After a summer of quarantine, like most I was looking forward to the starting of a new semester. Unfortunately, plans for the semester did not unfold as expected. However, I still progressed this semester in terms of learning about myself and the people around me. I stayed in an off-campus apartment complex during the duration of classes. I felt if I could not be on campus, I could at least be near the campus to feel as though I was at college. I brought my hobbies with me; my bike, my games, and I even had a little modelling station. As classes moved online, so too did my club NAMI. I am pleased to say I was elected vice president, and more importantly, that we maintained a healthy membership over the course of the semester. Some events NAMI was associated with over the semester concerned mental health discussions and panels. I felt as though I was ready to share my experience with others, and I contributed my perspective to two or three events. OSES also continued their probationary class, and I am slated to run shifts for spring 2021. I am looking forward to this especially as I can bring my knowledge into the field and help fellow students. COVID has exponentially increased an already existing mental health crisis amongst my generation. We must help each other if we want to curtail this issue let alone make it through the pandemic. Sometimes, all someone needs is a person to talk to them, to listen to them, and to empathize with them. I made several good friends in my apartment building over the course of the semester. They have been beneficial to my development, and I would likewise say I have been to theirs. I am grateful that despite the eventful start to the fall 2020 semester, I have progressed mentally with the help of my newfound friends and of course, my family.

We can all be our own worst enemy. Self-criticism is an act of sabotage against oneself. To an extent, it can be useful in developing yourself as a person, and I still engage in it. However, certain things are out of your control. During fall of 2019 I criticized myself for quandaries that I had no real control over. In large part, this issue occurred because my

OCD was running faster than I could keep up with it. Once I received help, and after some introspection, I began to catch up, and then surpass my mental dilemmas. I am by no means perfect, but I try my best, and I am not hard on myself as much as I was then. I ask you to likewise affirm your humanity and do not put yourself down. This pandemic has tested all of us. I acknowledge how this situation has been much more difficult for others, and as you read this perhaps it has been for you. People have lost loved ones, lost jobs, lost what has brought them joy. To that end I extend my sympathy. I want to say that we could easily fall into a trap of self-criticism because of these circumstances and due to the repetitious days of quarantine. At the end of the day, we can only try our best, whether that be in class or in life, and that is all that matters. In that vein, no one determines what your best is except you.

The idea of loneliness is especially prevalent now because of the pandemic. To be honest, this topic is difficult for me to address, but to reiterate the theme of the previous paragraph, I will try my best. The mind requires social stimulation. Even the most introverted of introverts require someone to speak to every now and again. You possibly were very extroverted before the pandemic, and the lack of social outlet has perhaps hit you hard especially. I can only offer advice based on my experience. I fulfill my alone time with hobbies, such as model building. There are numerous hobbies one can engage in, if funds are an issue, then watching videos on the hobby is an option. Sometimes I find myself watching my hobbies more than doing them. Other times, I like to read articles that pique my interest as I am always eager to learn something new, however inconsequential. As for social engagement, I talk with who I can when I can. Part of being a transfer student is not really knowing anyone. I used to be worried about reaching out to people because of this issue, however I have since realized this is no longer a problem and is more a benefit. Every person I talk to and meet is a fresh perspective in my life, and whether that perspective is positive or negative, it adds to my overall worldview. Hence, I no longer doubt if I should reach out to acquaintances I have met in my travels or talk to new people that come my way. I believe now we all just want someone to talk to; the subjects of discussion are only secondary to the fortune of speaking with another person. I find a sort of irony in realizing the value of social engagement at a time when it is most difficult to obtain. Nevertheless, I do not let this deter me. We all have a way of maintaining relationships with those we can no longer see in person. For me, video chats have been a way to maintain a level of social activity. Text messaging is of course another possibility. However, I believe sending text messages can only go so far. Text messages lack the facets of human social engagement. You cannot see the person and they cannot see you. There is no indication of emotion or attachment to the conversation over text, unless directly noted from one person to another. Therefore, I would encourage you to engage in video chats to maintain contact with people. While not the same as an in-person conversation, it is the next best option. We are fortunate to have such technology at our fingertips, utilize it.

So, my reader, that summarizes the trials and tribulations of the last year and a half of my life. I started my time at Oneonta overwhelmed with a flurry of emotion. I was not sure what I should do so I intensified my study efforts. After this action failed to resolve the issues that stemmed from my OCD, I sought help and have now become less self-critical of myself. Now that I have learned to let myself live, I have become less isolated. COVID has complicated my situation, but I remain hopeful, and I try the best I can every day. Some days, my best varies, though I am not harsh on myself when that variation occurs. I thank you for taking the time to read my narrative and I wish you strength in these turbulent times.

Pandemic Diary

January 8, 2021

JULIA PERRONE

Since the very start of COVID I have seen all the people around me change. Some took the time during quarantine to improve while others let it destroy them. I, however, experienced both sides of the spectrum. I have learned a lot about myself with all the time I had on my hands. I learned that there is value in acceptance. It was hard to accept that fact that I wouldn't be able to have a normal college experience, or a prom, or a regular graduation ceremony. It was all so devastating to me and all I could do was throw myself a pity party. Until I finally accepted the situation the world is in right now. On the other side of the spectrum, I did let this get the best of me. Not being able to do the things I love outside really put a dent on my mental health. I lost a lot of ambition and started to forget the things that make me happy. The long nights watching the news struck a fear in me that I've never felt before in my life. There was a point in time where I thought there was no light at the end of the tunnel as thousands were dying and with no cure. I am a type 1 Diabetic which makes me even more likely to get ill if I were to get the coronavirus. I have never seen my mom more concerned for me. It was scary to think that if I were to get this horrid disease that I wouldn't make it. Now I know that's a bit morbid so I'll talk about some positives. I realized to enjoy the little things now and I cherish life to its full extent. A hug from a friend, a meal with your family, and the simple exchange of please and thank you are all such minuscule things. But they are so important, and the simple things are the key to happiness. Things that used to be important to me aren't any more, like shopping, makeup, and how I'm gonna get my crush to like me back. Materialistic things are not important, and nothing is more powerful than strong relationships between family and friends.

As COVID-19 semester #2 draws to a close . . .

January 12, 2021

SUSAN GOODIER

I cry when I watch the evening news, no matter how hard I try to be stoic. Everyone is dealing with such angst. The leadership is sorely lacking, the climate is fighting back against centuries of human exploitation, and incidents of racial and other kinds of injustice are manifest. No one is passing through this time unscathed.

Yet, every day there is also something to appreciate or even celebrate. Most of my students have stuck with me and are wrapping up a semester of learning they can be truly proud of. I am so proud of them. They have supported me and each other in ways that matter, not just for today, but for all the days to come. Quite a few students are expressing their eagerness for the Spring 2021 semester. They will emerge brighter and better from this. My colleagues from departments all over campus have found ways to support each other. It goes so much further than just doing their jobs.

People across the nation and the world have thought creatively about how we can connect across the borders the Pandemic has built. This semester, the Pulitzer Prize-winning author Deborah Blum visited my class and presented lots of images that didn't make it into her book, *The Poisoner's Handbook*. My students enjoyed the reading and being able to ask the author questions. In other classes we connected with scholars working on fascinating projects that serendipitously fit with our course materials. My partner shared his extensive knowledge of Native American women's pottery making, and we received special access to a documentary about Haudenosaunee women in our Native American Women's History course. We connected across the internet in ways that I hope we can modify in positive ways when we get to a post-Pandemic world.

I have had amazing opportunities to expand my own horizons as well. I have been learning the Lenape language online with a Munsee teacher living in Canada with students from around the nation and as far away as Australia. I remotely created a museum exhibit, Zoomed into a colleague's class at the University of Rhode Island, and presented at institutions in Utah and in several New York State sites. I have been involved with documentaries and panel presentations and programs with lots of interesting people. And I continue to listen in on numerous presentations on fascinating topics—the African American community displaced by the building of Central Park in New York City, pioneer women's lives during westward expansion, and fighting slavery and racial injustice—generated by experts from across the United States and outside its borders. I have even attended virtual cooking classes and exercise classes!

The human spirit cannot be quenched: we are unstoppable. We do what we have to do and then some. This does not in any way diminish the terrible tragedies so many people are facing right now and for which I cannot stop grieving. But it does assure me we are going to be okay—we are going to get through this and come out the better when it is over.

Pandemic diary

January 12, 2021

SHASHA WALLIS

During the fall, I moved to live on campus. I loved being on campus but the risk of COVID was so big and as everyone knows, spread quickly causing campus to shut down. I left as soon as I could and left most of my dorm decorations and such behind to come back for two weeks later. I packed all the clothes I could and all the essentials and schoolwork because I wasn't sure how long we'd be gone for. Before that, I loved being on campus, my friends and I had a little friend group that hung out and went to most meals together and even went for dinner in town. I got really close with one of my friends from home and spent most days and nights with her. Adjusting to life on campus wasn't too hard for me because it just kind of felt like a sophisticated summer camp with masks. I enjoyed the independence and freedom of being able to go wherever I wanted without having to tell anyone else. I miss campus and I wish we had gotten to spend more than 12 days there because it was just starting to feel like home.

I think most people my age would say they're angry or upset with the way COVID has taken away some events in our lives, but honestly, I'm a little thankful. My graduation still got to happen, and I didn't have to waste as much time sitting through the ceremony. Instead, I had a designated time to show up to walk the stage which made it much easier and quicker to finish the ceremony and get my diploma. I am a little upset I didn't get to play my senior season as captain of my rugby team, but I'm sure there will be other opportunities to make up for the lost time and season. I don't really mind wearing masks and honestly, it's the least we can do to protect everyone else from ourselves, but a lot of people seem to have a problem with it. I think a lot of people forget that this isn't the end of the world and there have been pandemics that society has survived before and continued afterwards. I believe people should take this time, if they haven't already to reflect on what they want and how they treat others going forward. Isolation is the perfect place for reevaluation and realignment within oneself.

Personally, for me the pandemic has been a gift. I had a rough year going on before that, I was dealing with the repercussions of my parents' separation, the betrayal of a close friend, and the death of my childhood best friend. Before that I wasn't coping well and lack of sleep from school was not helping me heal any faster. Instead, I'd be overtired and unmotivated, falling asleep in class, and when I got home, I would feel alone and unresolved from all the changes happening in my life. So, when the pandemic happened, I was finally able to rest and catch up on months' worth of sleep. Once I recovered from overexhaustion, I could finally see the problems I was facing instead of ignoring them. In my isolation I realized a lot of self-worth and did a lot of much needed healing and reconciliation with myself and those I'd pushed away or unintentionally hurt. So, while the pandemic did take many things away, it made me a better person and I think that's more important than anything temporary like senior year or anything that us freshmen missed out on.

Vaccinated!

January 15, 2021

Matthew C. Hendley

January 15, 2021 will be a day I will always remember. It is the day that I received my first dose of the Moderna COVID vaccine. I drove up to the Otsego Board of Health Meadows complex near Cooperstown on a misty morning past snow-covered fields. Once I got there, things moved smoothly. The staff were kind and efficient. The shot was painless. I would love to be able to say that as I drove back the sun broke through, the mist parted, and the world shone in brilliant upstate New York winter sunshine. However, that didn't happen. It was still a grey morning. The mist dissipated slightly, and I arrived back at my office. I spent the rest of the day working, albeit with a slightly sore left arm.

Still—I could not get over the fact that I had finally been vaccinated. As I am scheduled to teach an in-person section of a class in the Spring semester, I was eligible. I am the first in my immediate family to reach this milestone. I still need a second dose. I still need to be careful. However, I have been vaccinated.

Vaccination. It is just a word. However, after what my family, the nation and the world have been through in the last year it seems to mean so much more.

Vaccination. It hints at new possibilities and a return to a more normal way of existence: A life without masks. A life with actual human interactions. A life with travel. A life that includes going out to the movies, sharing meals with my friends at each other's houses and all the other small human pleasures that make life worth living. A life that is not under constant threat of extinction. A life without so much suffering and death.

I dearly hope that once all my family is vaccinated that we can actually cross the border into Canada and visit with parents, siblings, nephews, nieces, in-laws, and friends whom we have not seen since summer 2019. I dearly hope that once vaccinations ramp up, my college can return to its usual routine of in-person teaching, student activities, visiting speakers, etc. I dearly hope that we can put the pandemic year into the rearview mirror and think about living again.

On November 10, 1942, following almost three years of constant setbacks, the British secured their first major military victory over the German Army at the Battle of El Alamein in Egypt. To mark this occasion, Winston Churchill said the following in a speech at the Lord Mayor's luncheon in London—"Now this is not the end. It is not even the beginning of the end. But it is, perhaps, the end of the beginning." The Second World War still had several years to run to its course but at that moment, hope in victory finally appeared.

It is my fondest wish that January 2021 marks the end of the beginning. I finally have hope that victory over COVID can be secured, however long the battle may be.

Proud to be a naturalized U.S. citizen

January 20, 2021

Maria Cristina Montoya

Today, January 20, 2021, was full of symbolism, pride, and hope. Twenty-five years ago, I had sworn to the flag of the United States of America to respect and contribute to this country, my second home. Back then I felt obligated, committed, and compromised by the possibility of opportunity; however, my heart was still nostalgic for the land south that raised my consciousness, still did not see me mature.

I have matured surrounded by good people, honest and loyal U.S. Americans. As an immigrant, and outsider, I only noticed division of the union and the principles that thread this democratic project in recent years. I feared discrimination and the social nightmare that most of us escaped when we decided to cross the border. I even suffered through the idea I had to leave again; I am too old for another exile journey. But today, after a day of symbolism, and a final happy episode, I feel immense gratitude by having earned a piece of land in the north, with water, a family, and surrounded by good people, "hombres y mujeres de bien."

Today, I am of a positive mind, and this pandemic is just a "shake" to our hearts that shows us humans, how fragile yet resilient we are when we need to survive. Today, I finally understand my oath to the U.S. American Flag.

Part V

Spring 2021

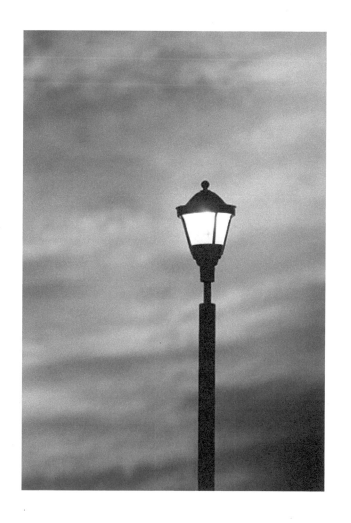

12

February 2021

SUNY ONEONTA

February 3—Presidential Search Committee officially begins search for new SUNY Oneonta president.

February 15—*Chronicle of Higher Education* publishes an article highlighting SUNY Oneonta's response to COVID pandemic in spring 2020 and fall 2020.

ONEONTA

February 12—National Baseball Hall of Fame cancels Classic Weekend in May and scales back July induction.

February 24—Otsego County sees surge in cases with forty-one positives (twenty-eight of whom were students from SUNY Oneonta and Hartwick College).

NEW YORK

February 3—Governor Cuomo announces vaccinations to be given at Yankee Stadium mass vaccination site.

February 15—All adults with certain underlying conditions became eligible for vaccinations. Qualifying conditions included cancer, moderate to severe asthma, obesity, and hypertension.

USA

February 1—More Americans vaccinated than infected with COVID-19.

February 12—United States purchases 200 million Moderna and Pfizer Vaccines.

February 26—Fifty million COVID-19 vaccine doses administered.

February 27—FDA grants emergency use authorization for Johnson and Johnson Vaccine.

WORLD

February 24—Global COVAX initiative to ensure equitable access to vaccines begins. First delivery made to Ghana.

Diarios en pandemia

February 16, 2021

Nicole Barreca

Cuando la pandemia llegó por primera vez a mi país, no pensé que fuera real. Estaba muy confundida por lo que era porque no había pasado por algo como esto antes. Me di cuenta de que era serio cuando pasaron 6 meses y las cosas solo estaban empeorando: ver gente caminando con máscaras, asustada de acercarse a otros, usando desinfectante de manos y con guantes donde quiera que iban y mirándote extraño si estornudabas—se convirtió en nuestra nueva normalidad. No recuerdo cómo es ir a clases en persona, ir a la biblioteca o la unión para comprar un café y hablar con amigos, o hablar con los estudiantes y profesores cara a cara en la clase, es difícil despertar cada día sabiendo que haré exactamente lo mismo que hice el día anterior. Mis días parecen ser muy repetitivos y no emocionantes, desearía poder volver a tiempos anteriores a la pandemia para terminar mis años universitarios. Mirar mi computadora todos los días durante todo el día ha sido muy agotador y me hace sentir como un zombi. Me siento muy decepcionada y frustrada porque la mitad de mi tercer año aquí y todo mi último año se está desarrollando de esta manera, y que no podré cruzar el escenario en la graduación frente a mi familia y todos mis profesores. Es difícil vivir en estos tiempos con 21 años, pero seguiré tratando de ser lo más positivo que pueda a medida que avancen los días.

When the pandemic first came to my country, I didn't think it was real. I was very confused about what it was because I hadn't been through something like this before. I realized it was serious when 6 months passed and things were only getting worse—seeing people walking around in masks, scared to approach others, using hand sanitizer and gloves wherever they go, and looking weird at you if you sneeze—it became our new normal. I don't remember what it's like to go to class in person, go to the library or the union building to buy coffee and talk with friends, or talk to students and teachers face to face in class, it is difficult to wake up each day knowing that I will do exactly the same as I did the day before. My days seem to be very repetitive and not exciting; I wish I could go back to pre-pandemic times to finish my college years. Looking at my computer every day for the whole day has been very tiring and makes me feel like a zombie. I feel very disappointed and frustrated that half of my junior year here and my entire senior year is unfolding in this way, and that I won't be able to cross the stage at graduation in front of my family and all my professors. It's hard to live in these times at 21, but I'll keep trying to be as positive as I can as the days go on.

13

March 2021

SUNY ONEONTA

March 18—Mass public vaccination site opened at SUNY Oneonta.

ONEONTA

March 5—Of 147 COVID positives recorded in the last ten days in Otsego County, 47 percent are reported to be from college students and employees.

NEW YORK

March 5—Governor Cuomo announced event, arts, and entertainment venues can reopen at 33 percent capacity (with a limit of 100 people indoors or 200 outdoors) starting April 2.

March 10—New York residents aged sixty or older became eligible for vaccination as well as public-facing government and nonprofit employees starting March 17.

March 11—Governor Cuomo announces domestic travelers will not have to quarantine when arriving from out of state starting April 1.

March 29—New York State lowers vaccine age eligibility to thirty.

USA

March 1—Johnson and Johnson Vaccine rollout begins.

March 3—President Biden promises vaccines will be available for every US adult by May.

March 25—President Biden announces new vaccine goal of 200 million doses in his first 100 days in office.

WORLD

March 17—Vaccine doses expected to reach 700 million by summer.

March 20—World Health Organization approves Johnson and Johnson vaccine for global emergency use and COVAX initiative.

A COVID Coda to Baby Yoda
(and wild turkeys for good measure)

March 2, 2021

Matthew C. Hendley

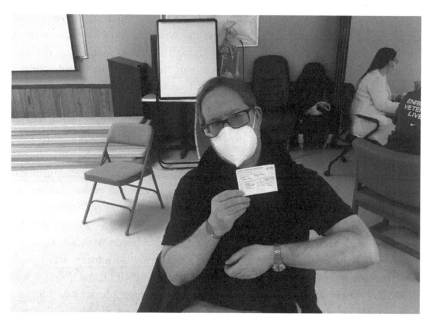

Posing after receiving my second vaccination: After my encounter with the wild turkeys but before meeting Baby Yoda!

It is perhaps befitting an extremely weird year that my final blog entry should revolve around wild turkeys and Baby Yoda. Though at first not obvious soulmates, these types of creatures do fit together in the menagerie of my mind as revealed during my second vaccination and immediately thereafter between February 16–17, 2021.

I will lay it all out for you.

The wild turkeys were unexpected. On February 16, I was duly driving up Otsego County Road 33 on my way to the Otsego County Meadows complex for my second Moderna vaccination. Having had my first vaccination without major side effects a month before and with the weather relatively clear for a February morning in upstate New York, I had few concerns. I was driving the sole car on a country road approaching my destination with a set goal in mind. I was listening to NPR. My second vaccination would put me on the path to immunity. I could teach the in-person part of my dual modality class with confidence. I would be protected from this awful disease and a life of normality beckoned. Which of course is where the wild turkeys came in.

Let me assure you, gentle reader, that when a middle-aged professor is carefully driving below the legal speed limit up a country road towards a medical rendezvous the last thing, he expects is a flock of not so bright birds sitting on the road. Now don't get me wrong. I have a certain respect for the glory of the American turkey. Though raised in Canada, I partook of turkey dinners for Canadian Thanksgiving (celebrated in October but I digress). I eagerly adapted to American Thanksgiving and have eaten my fill of this fine bird for the November celebration. However, I was less than thrilled to see them sitting on County Road 33 without a care in the world. I cursed, hit the brake to slow down further, swerved ever so slightly and that did the trick. I avoided turkey catastrophe. The ungainly birds slowly took flight one after the other and thankfully avoided making communion with my windshield. I was safe and so were they. I did reflect briefly on the historical claim that Benjamin Franklin recommended the turkey as the official symbol of the United States rather than the bald eagle. However, I got over it. I got my second Moderna shot and drove home without incident.

Which brings me to Baby Yoda. The second vaccination went well. My arm did not hurt as much as after the first one (minimal Tylenol was needed). I wisely took the next day off from major work duties and thought I would do some academic reading or light work around the house. Boy was I wrong. My brain felt mentally foggy (though I guess my wife and work colleagues would say that was only slightly different from my brain on most days). To be accurate my brain felt MORE mentally foggy than usual. My arm throbbed a bit. However, I was tired. What better way to spend the day than to lie on the couch and watch streaming of "The Mandalorian"? Which I did. I had been meaning to watch it for ages but have been too busy. As my brain drifted in and out of naps, I had some incredibly lucid dreams. I also met Baby Yoda on screen. Small, green, and wise, Baby Yoda was the polar opposite of those stupid turkeys that I almost collided with the day before. Baby Yoda endured numerous adventures, briefly revealed the powers of "the Force" and ran off with the Mandalorian's main character (a bounty hunter who has a fit of remorse) for safer pastures. What could be better?

In closing I hope to see much more of Baby Yoda in the future. I also hope never to see a wild turkey again.

I am coming back to my classroom!

March 5, 2021

Maria Cristina Montoya

You stayed your entire life in college,
PhD Requirement.
Done with taking exams.
But eternal HW: grading to do.
I am coming back to my classroom.
Masked until we are all immunized.

Autobiography, Vocation and Pandemic

March 11, 2021

Miguel León

One of the most positive aspects of quarantining during this pandemic is that it has forced us to find new ways to communicate with others using alternative means. One is via virtual calls. Constant communication via virtual calls is, in and of itself, representative of a new era of communication. You discover new ways of talking to your parents, your family, friends, colleagues, coworkers, etc. New topics have emerged which is a pleasant surprise. Before the pandemic, I started a new project: writing an academic autobiography about my life as a professional historian. These virtual conversations have provided me with a lot of new material for my autobiography by listening to family and friends talking about their lives and common experiences and has taught me so many new things about remembering and selective memories.

A crucial part of my autobiographical reflections is related to my interest in regional history of Peru. One of the most important sources of inspiration for my decision to become a historian was to study the history of the regions of my ancestors, these two are: Huánuco and the Conchucos region. During the pandemic, I was invited twice to share my research on these regions via virtual talks. I was happily surprised by the new things I learned through these talks and the audience's feedback.

First, I did not know that I had a larger audience. With FaceBook Live I was able to learn that approximately 600 people were interested to see my talk. Some of these people, who live in small towns and even small Andean communities in Peru, followed my bibliography and asked very specific questions about my books. I remember early in my career traveling to these regions and small towns with the desire to share my findings. It seems that now that I live 3,650 miles away, I discovered a new way to reach them.

Second, one of the talks I gave was about the value of the documents of the Regional Archives of Huánuco. This talk was very personal because I heard recollections from workers of this archive and memories that they had about me as a young historian. Empathy was not one of my virtues during that time of my life. During the 1980s, to support myself I had to work my last two years of college, so I conducted my research during vacations. In one of my visits to the archives of Huánuco, I was not too happy to lose a half day of research because the workers of the archive were celebrating "Archivist Day," and I complained about it.

Thirty years after that moment no one has forgotten my behavior and made humorous remarks about it today. Yes, I was very passionate about reading the documents, discovering new things every day, waking up in the morning and knowing that the documents were going to provide me with another piece of the puzzle that I was solving. Now I laugh at myself, and I celebrate the fact that even though I was a bit intolerant as a young historian, the workers of the archive remember it with a mixture of scandalous joy.

During 1997 and 1998 I did archival work in the Huánuco archives for my dissertation. Thanks to Columbia University and other institutions I was able to spend several months working in these archives. The Director, Deomar Hidalgo (rest in peace, unfortunately he died in a car accident a few years ago) was especially supportive of my work. While doing research, I talked to him about my research agendas and listened to him talk about his plans of cataloging and indexing colonial documents. I finished my dissertation in 1999 and published it as a book in 2002. I went back to Huánuco as a SUNY professor many years later. In one of the many conversations, he sounded a bit frustrated with the fact that I now live in New York, and I have many time constraints because I always had to return back to the USA. "Why did you move so far, Miguel?" he asked me. I was caught by surprise and could not answer. He did not wait for an answer. I still don't know how to answer that question completely, but I guess I found in New York a place to work well as a historian of regions of Peru despite that enormity of the distance. The pandemic, although horrific and cruel, has taught me that no matter the distance we can still continue to communicate, learn, and support one another.

Seven

March 14, 2021

ANN TRAITOR

Seven.

For many people, seven is a lucky, fun number. Seven wonders of the World! Snow White and the Seven Dwarfs! Three sevens for the slot machine jackpot!

For me, seven is none of those things. Seven is the number of people I have lost due to COVID.

It started in the final week of last March and continued with frightening regularity over the ensuing nine months. Death seemed to stalk me. I started to dread looking at my email or getting a phone call from a relative. For whom is "Death" the last friend now, escorting my loved ones away?

The first one was the hardest. The shock factor really hit home. My work kept me sane. I buried myself in books and worked to keep my mind off of the loss, off of the lack of the funeral, off of the idea that the ashes were in a can in a "holding room," waiting to be picked up at some future, unspecified time. I told myself that others have it worse, be grateful for what still remains.

But the numbers piled up. The phone kept ringing. Often the end came so quickly that the phone call related the scary trip to the hospital, the valiant efforts by medical professionals, and the excruciating end, all in one breathless statement. I started to mourn quickly, speeding through the process, not really letting any of it settle in for fear I would not be able to cope.

This past weekend marked the one-year anniversary of COVID—the lockdowns, the fear, the death. In the chill of early March, as the evening settled in, I sat outside, alone in the woods. I remembered all those who have left me, and I cried, and I cried, and I cried.

Pandemic workout

March 14, 2021

Michelle Hendley

"You can do a workout with a N95 mask?" asked my friend as we passed each other in front of the entrance to the large gym at the local YMCA. I am not sure if he was in awe or incredulous because his expression was hidden behind his surgical mask. "It's not an N95 mask. It's a KN95 mask and yeah, I can," I replied.

Doing high-impact aerobics with a mask is certainly a better alternative to what I had been doing since the beginning of the pandemic when the YMCA temporarily closed its doors. Attending my Thursday evening fitness class has been an important ritual for several years and it became even more essential in the early days of the COVID-19 crisis. As a result of the pandemic, class was now on my iPad with my instructor, dear friend, and library colleague, Kim, leading her students via Zoom. My classmates were dots on my screen. My workout space was now in the guest room in my house. The room nicknamed "the man cave," is roomy enough for guests but a tad confined for a workout.

I am very grateful that Kim continued the class virtually. Her weekly workout helped me to cope with my day-to-day normal stress and elevated, pandemic related anxiety. Nonetheless, I missed her in-person positive energy, the camaraderie of the other members of class, and the spacious fitness room. Looking at a small iPad screen was becoming challenging. And after a long day of work-related Teams' meetings, spending time on Zoom for exercise was less than ideal. Despite this, the alternative, not attending Zoom aerobics, was an unviable option.

Thankfully, aerobics and other fitness classes, with very strict protocols, resumed at the YMCA in the summer. I leapt at the opportunity to return to in-person aerobics. No more iPad! No more Zoom! No more dots! No more confined man cave! That being said, I was now required to adapt to the many rules associated with pandemic era, in-person fitness instruction: class size is limited, pre-registration is compulsory, social distancing is oblig-atory, and mask wearing is mandatory.

Wearing a mask during the workout is not without its challenges. The mask makes my face hot and irritates my skin. Breathing can be tricky. Nevertheless, these inconveniences are worthwhile because I can exercise in a spacious, well-ventilated facility with my instructor and fellow participants.

Recently, as I was about to enter the Y's gym for class, I overheard another member expressing his fatigue with wearing a mask. He was so tired of it. I empathize with him; however, when the choice is between exercising virtually on Zoom without a mask or exercising in-person with a mask, I choose in-person with a mask.

I didn't check to see how many people died yesterday

March 15, 2021

Ed Beck

In November I wrote that I was constantly doomscrolling. I was obsessed with looking at numbers, trends, maps, risk levels. I said I didn't check the weather outside because I didn't go outside anyway.

I know the pandemic isn't over. I know that just because I have received my first vaccine I still need to mask up, follow social distancing. But I can't help but feel that a weight has been lifted from my mind. It's not quite hope I'm feeling, but an absence of constant dread. When I look back at this pandemic diary project, what I think about most are the posts I didn't write, when I was too overwhelmed to put anything together.

- Early in the Pandemic, I really struggled with my chronic migraines. I had a migraine that would not go away, and I ended up in the emergency room because no other doctor would see me including my doctor or the urgent care. The ER staff was amazing, but it was frustrating that no one else would see me.

- Later, one of my friends had an uncle die from COVID-19. At a time when the pandemic seemed to be something that was happening to other people, it was my first connection to someone who died of the disease.

- When my own uncle got the disease, I couldn't bring myself to write about it. He is fine now, but it very easily could have gone the other way with his other conditions.

- When my aunt died of cancer, I was angry that she spent time in pain and alone in the hospital because of limited visiting. I still feel like I don't have closure because my family couldn't gather and grieve.

The Semester of Living Dangerously has helped me through all of this. Even when I couldn't write myself, it helped to know that other people were feeling the same things. The entries of other people captured my feelings even when I couldn't write them myself.

14

April 2021

SUNY ONEONTA

April 29—Students have one more week to be pool-tested for COVID-19 before leaving for the summer break.

ONEONTA

April 2—Senator Charles Schumer meets with community leaders to discuss priorities and opportunities in the region.

NEW YORK

April 2—Residents sixteen years old and older are now eligible for the COVID-19 vaccine.

April 27—Fully vaccinated individuals no longer have to wear masks in public, outdoor spaces.

April 29—All state-run vaccination centers are open for walk-in appointments.

USA

April 2—Almost 40 percent of the country's adults have been vaccinated.

April 24—The total number of COVID-19 cases surpasses 32 million.

WORLD

April 5—Brazil surpasses 13 million COVID-19 cases.

Three things I learned about SUNY Oneonta

April 18, 2021

Maria Cristina Montoya

Talk to incoming class fall 2021

Good evening, I am Maria Cristina Montoya and I have been teaching in the Foreign Languages and Literatures Department since the new millennium started.

Allow me to re-create for you the three most important things I have learned about Oneonta:

First,

We are a community that cares, helps each other, collaborates, recovers, and starts again.

I learned this in the classroom:

1. by observing my students' diverse learning styles.

2. with my colleagues who collaborated to switch gears and teach fully online within a one-week time frame.

3. with the entire institution by powering multiple TEAMS of us to plan, to act, to recover and to start again.

Second,
We are all about traditions.
Let me give you my three favorite traditions:

1. Before pandemic times, every fall, first day of classes we had an opening brunch in the middle of the quad. All students, faculty, and employees ate and chatted together. It was exciting to see everyone back and eager to learn and to experience. It was really like a college carnival. I wish for that to happen again, after the pandemic, when we all may eat together in a large group.

2. Ice cream for freshmen after passing through the pillars. It signifies their entrance into the four years of a "roller coaster ride" of their undergraduate education where they discover a lot of themselves, grow and become critical thinkers with coherent arguments to state their positions about themselves in the world. During the motivational clapping as they walk down to the quad, they all look like toddlers to me. This year I will have one of my own in the crowd, an Oneonta Native.

3. Champagne for seniors as they pass the pillars on their way out into the "real world." This happens every graduation eve, and I do not miss the opportunity to celebrate with a drink to my graduates. I also collect the fancy champagne glasses that are given to keep. I cry and clap on that day, all of them are my own.

Third,

On April 4th, 2000, during my job interview, I learned that Oneonta was the place I wanted to grow.

And "Ay Dios" if I have grown:

1. I grew a family, counting six members now, and an immigrant adopted dog from Colombia.

2. I grew a career in higher education:

   • I learned to engage my students.

   • I learned to challenge them to be creative and critical thinkers.

   • I learned to guide them to be successful and passionate in all they do.

- I learned to master ideas, to propose and create fun applied learning experiences for my students, for example:

  - Collaborative Online International learning, connecting my classroom to another classroom in the world.

  - Faculty led-off courses abroad with students and faculty colleagues. I have done five of them and the adrenaline that runs through my blood during these experiences is hard to describe, I am mesmerized when I see their eyes upon discoveries.

  - International faculty partnerships to enhance and diversify our teaching practice.

  - Community outreach through the Multicultural Community Center, where students volunteer hours to serve local, national, and international communities by teaching languages and assisting children with any academic need—more important now, during pandemic, when we are all learning online.

  - Creativity in research and digital innovative projects owned by students and networked with Oneonta alumni, such as the "Living Bilingual Blog."

There are a lot more examples that each faculty at Oneonta offers to engage our students.

And lastly,

1. I aged happily going to work. I must be thankful of my privilege. I am a lucky human being who loves to wake up every dawn, at 4 a.m., to work. It is true, so if you are a student in my class, and sleep with your phone ON beside your bed, I will wake you up before the sun, with my daily announcements or reminders.

There are three things I learned about SUNY Oneonta:

1. We are a community.

2. We value traditions.

3. It is the place where I chose to grow.

15

May–June 2021

May 2021

SUNY ONEONTA

May 16—The campuswide mask policy remains unchanged.

ONEONTA

May 4—The City of Oneonta announces it will close Main Street in order to send off the college graduates.

NEW YORK

May 10—Outdoor social gathering limit expanded from 200 to 500 people.

May 26—Governor Cuomo announces a vaccine-incentive program that offers a full scholarship to any New York State public college or university, chosen by random draw.

USA

May 13—The CDC says fully vaccinated individuals do not need to wear masks in most situations.

May 29—Massachusetts rescinds most of its COVID-19 restrictions.

WORLD

May 26—India surpasses 27 million COVID-19 cases and 300,000 deaths.

June 2021

SUNY ONEONTA

June 3—Faculty, staff, and students can now host visitors on campus and inside buildings.

June 22—Fully vaccinated faculty and staff no longer need to wear masks or undergo weekly testing.

ONEONTA

June 18—Gov. Andrew Cuomo announces that the mass vaccination site at SUNY Oneonta would close on June 21.

NEW YORK STATE

June 25—With the New York State Travel Advisory no longer in effect, travelers arriving in New York no longer have to submit traveler health forms.

USA

June 21—The CDC reports that more than 45 percent of all Americans are fully vaccinated, with 1.1 million doses per day given.

June 29—The Delta variant accounts for 26 percent of all COVID-19 cases in the US. Weekly cases of COVID in children are down to 8,400, the lowest since May 2020.

WORLD

June 29—The World Health Organization reports that the number of weekly deaths worldwide continues to decrease. However, the number of new weekly cases did increase in African, European, and Eastern Mediterranean regions.

Languishing through my walk-in closet museum

June 7, 2021

Maria Cristina Montoya

Main Gallery

Boots, no recollection when last exhibited. Almost forgot these existed.
Fancy summer shoes, all acquired for the collection "Summer 2019."
NEGRO, MARRÓN CLARO, CAFÉ, ROJO, ROSADO, AMARILLO,
ANARANJADO, AZUL, VERDE, MORADO Y BLANCO.
Dresses, Blouses, Jackets . . . All still. Reminders of moments when these
were displayed.

Down Gallery

Pants, unassessed since March 2020; some will be heading to other collections, at other museums.

Season Gallery

Luggage, empty, in good condition.
Extraño la vida antes de la Pandemia.

An Archive for All

Mass Observation as the Inspiration for the Blog and the Book

Matthew C. Hendley and Ann A. Traitor

Introduction

It almost sounds like the beginning of a joke: a poet, an ornithologist, and a documentary filmmaker meet in an apartment in London to discuss how to uncover the collective unconscious. Rather than delivering a punch line, these three men were laying the foundations for an exciting experiment which came to be called Mass Observation.

The men met in 1936, during the "Abdication Crisis" in which Edward VIII gave up the Crown in order to marry the American divorcee, Wallis Simpson. According to the many newspaper column inches devoted to the crisis, the British people feared for the future of the monarchy and the future of their empire. One letter in particular caught the eyes of our three men. The letter was written by Geoffrey Pyke and had been printed in the December 12, 1936 issue of the *New Statesman*, a political and cultural magazine. In his letter to the *New Statesman*, Geoffrey Pyke reflected on the Abdication Crisis, the press, and the public reaction:

> How far the press reflected, and how far it evoked and molded public opinion during the last ten days it is impossible to say. Thousands of letters have poured into the offices of newspapers and other organizations from obscure and eminent people alike.

It is most important that these should be preserved and made accessible.

It would seem that the majority of the inhabitants of the Empire are unable to tolerate the image of a Queen—whose chief function together with her Consort would be to be an object of idolization—who has previously been married to two men who are still alive. . . . It will help our understanding and sensible behavior towards this if we have obtained in some measure an understanding of our own recent psychopathic reactions.[1]

One of our three men, the poet Charles Madge, answered Mr. Pyke's call for an "anthropology of ourselves" in a letter of January 2, 1937, where Madge wrote his memorable phrase that "only mass observers can create mass science."[2] There was already a group of people engaged in this very activity of "observing," and Madge encouraged anyone and everyone to volunteer. Madge's friend, the documentary filmmaker, Humphrey Jennings, was already on board. The ornithologist Tom Harrisson read Madge's letter in the Bolton Public Library. Noting the invitation at the bottom and wishing to join Madge's group, Harrisson contacted Madge. Shortly thereafter, all three men met in an apartment in London to discuss how to uncover the collective unconscious.

The result of that meeting in London was a third letter to the *New Statesman*, this time introducing their new organization to the public: "Mass Observation." Noting that the abdication crisis was the touch paper for their idea, the authors ambitiously wrote that "Mass Observation develops out of anthropology, psychology, and the sciences which study man—but it plans to work with a mass of observers. Already we have fifty observers at work on two sample problems."[3] Their enthusiasm in those heady, early days was palpable as they hoped for 5,000 volunteer observers who would grapple with such questions from the topical ("behavior of people at war memorials" and "the private lives of midwives") to the unusual ("bathroom behavior" and "funerals and undertakers") to the bizarre ("beards, armpits, eyebrows").[4]

---

1. As quoted in Dorothy Sheridan, Brian Street, and David Bloome, *Writing Ourselves: Mass-Observation and Literacy Practices* (Cresshill, NJ: Hampton Press, 2000), 22–23.

2. As quoted in Sheridan, Street, and Bloome, *Writing Ourselves*, 24.

3. As quoted in Sheridan, Street, and Bloome, *Writing Ourselves*, 25.

4. As quoted in Sheridan, Street, and Bloome, *Writing Ourselves*, 25.

The Birth of Mass Observation

Once Mass Observation (MO) was officially launched, it set up two distinct units that revealed the extremely contradictory approaches taken by the project's main founders. The first unit, headed by Tom Harrisson, was located in the northern Lancashire mill town of Bolton. It specialized in direct observation by participant observers. The second unit, headed by Charles Madge and assisted by Humphrey Jennings, was based in London, and specialized in written observation by indirect observers. Together they provided a new way of looking at Britain and left a remarkable record of primary source documents and published work that historians are still mulling over decades later. Between 1937 and 1940, Harrisson and his team of up to sixty observers lived among the population of Bolton (which he called Worktown). Eventually joined by Charles Madge, the team assiduously observed every possible phenomenon, including religion, politics, housing, saving and spending and leisure, associational life, sexual habits, and so on.[5] Some of their most colorful material came out of their leisure investigations, which took them to pubs, gambling dens, the cinema, dance halls, wrestling matches, and the nearby Blackpool seaside resort.[6] Harrisson would return to Bolton after the war with some of the same team to write a retrospective work titled *Britain Revisited*.

Being a poet rather than a swashbuckling adventurer, it is perhaps unsurprising that Madge's approach was different. Based in Blackheath in northern London, Madge's team began to compile detailed written observations by individual diary writers. Their approach with MO was to enlist a number of volunteer correspondents (called the National Panel) who would regularly write in journals that would be sent in to the Blackheath headquarters. The writings would be guided by instructions called "directives." Beginning in February 1937, they began to record everything that happened to them on the twelfth day of every month in the run-up to the coronation of George VI on May 12, 1937. In time this would be expanded to a host of other topics that the observers would write about, guided by new monthly directives. The period from 1937 to 1945 was filled with tumultuous national events and wrenching social changes. During that time 1,095 people would

5. Judith Heimann, *The Most Offending Soul Alive: Tom Harrisson and His Remarkable Life* (Honolulu: University of Hawai'i Press, 1998), 132.

6. Angus Calder and Dorothy Sheridan (ed.), *Speak for Yourself: A Mass-Observation Anthology, 1937–49* (London: Jonathan Cape, 1984), 247.

be part of the National Panel, though at its peak in 1939 only five men and one woman replied dutifully to every single directive.[7]

Unfortunately, the first major publication jointly authored by Madge and Jennings was a bit of a mess. *May the Twelfth* was a 400-page opus assembled from the surveys sent in from the twelfth of every month between February and May 1937. *May the Twelfth* was supposed to be the antidote to press speculation about public opinion. However, as a written work it is a failure, and some critics like Samuel Hynes have said it is "unreadable."[8] Harrisson hated *May the Twelfth*, and noted in a 1938 letter, "it was a crazy idea to have it edited by a whole bunch of intellectual poets."[9] He took a firmer hand in future publications and Jennings left the core team of Mass Observation. Spurred on by Harrison, MO published two much more readable books in 1938–39—*First Year's Work* and *Britain by Mass-Observation*.

First Year's Work is a short and somewhat breezy book that introduces readers to the Mass Observation project and elucidates some initial investigations into key components of working-class life such as smoking, pubs, football pools, and holiday excursions to Blackpool seaside resort. Based on the feedback gathered from observers, MO was able to note that both smoking and beer drinking were engaged in mostly for social factors and that widespread betting in football pools revealed not only greed but a way of sustaining hope.[10] Insightful criticism to *First Year's Work* is found in the afterword titled "A Nationwide Intelligence Service" by Bronislaw Malinowski. Malinowski, a renowned professor of Anthropology at the University of London, was impressed with the concept behind MO and the passion of

---

7. Calder and Sheridan, *Speak for Yourself*, 73.

8. As Hynes acidly but perceptively notes of *May the Twelfth*, "The materials are documentary, the presentation is literary, and the classifying and analysing are polemical; the book attempts to be at once scientific and political, to be comprehensive and yet readable, to record and make judgements. In the end it fails, it becomes unreadable, but not because of the politics of the literariness; what kills it, finally is the flat repetitiousness of the observers' reports—it is the mass [*sic*] in the Mass-Observation that is numbing," Samuel Hynes, *The Auden Generation: Literature and Politics in England in the 1930s* (New York: Viking, 1972), 286.

9. Tom Harrisson to Geoffrey Gorer (1938) as cited in the Afterword by David Pocock in Humphrey Jennings and Charles Madge (eds.) *May the Twelfth—Mass-Observation Day-Surveys by over two hundred observers* (London: Faber and Faber, 1987 [rpt.]). Originally published in 1937, 418.

10. Charles Madge and Tom Harrisson (eds.), *First Year's Work 1937–38 by Mass Observation* (London: Lindsay Drummond, 1938), 22–23; 37.

its creators. However, he strongly argued. "Despite all its promise and the value of its results, it needs a thorough overhaul of principle and method."[11] Malinowski called for a reduced staff of trained informants and the need for a much more scientific approach when it came to collecting and categorizing the information that it gathered. His criticisms would be echoed by social science critics of MO. One unkind writer from 1937 claimed that Mass Observation was "scientifically, about as valuable, as a chimpanzee's tea party at the zoo." Nevertheless, Mass Observation persisted.[12]

Britain by Mass-Observation was their most impactful prewar publication. It appeared as a mass market paperback Penguin special in 1939 and sold over 100,000 copies in ten days.[13] Following the pattern from *First Year's Work*, *Britain by Mass-Observation* once again dived into working-class life to look at attitudes toward democracy, free-style wrestling, home life, religion, and culture. Its two most important sections were on two very different topics—a dance craze known as the Lambeth Walk and the Munich Crisis of 1938. The book's most insightful analysis of the public response was to the Munich crisis, which arose from Hitler's claims to the Sudetenland in 1938.[14] For the ten days at the height of the crisis, MO observers were able to take apart how the British people felt. Two very important points picked up include the fact that there was a strong split among working-class people interviewed by MO of men against Neville Chamberlain and women in support of him. It also pointed out that public revulsion against the Munich deal (which betrayed and dismembered Czechoslovakia but avoided a new world war) grew quickly in the days after it and that press image of public relief and near hysteria in support for Chamberlain in the deal's aftermath was overblown.[15]

Through these prewar publications and the unpublished records MO accumulated, the organization played a vital role in trying to explain interwar Britain to its own citizens and leave key archival records for future historians.

---

11. Bronislow Malinowski, "A Nationwide Intelligence Service," in Madge and Harrisson, *First Year's Work*, 87.

12. Annebella Pollen, "Research Methodology in Mass Observation Past and Present: 'Scientifically, about as Valuable as a Chimpanzee's Tea Party at the Zoo'?," *History Workshop Journal*, 75 (Spring 2013): 213.

13. Angus Calder, "Introduction," in Tom Harrisson and Charles Madge, *Britain by Mass-Observation* (London: Cresset Library, 1986). Originally published in 1939, vii.

14. Heimann, *Most Offending Soul Alive*, 148.

15. Harrisson and Madge, *Britain by Mass Observation*, 242–45.

Mass Observation Goes to War

If the Munich crisis showed the value of Mass Observation to record public opinion over a limited period during a diplomatic crisis, the Second World War gave MO semiofficial status with the government and left a priceless treasure trove of wartime records for future historians.

By September 1939, Tom Harrisson had returned to London and was now in charge of the National Panel. The government soon understood that MO had particular advantages and talents in monitoring public opinion that the less agile government ministries lacked. In 1940, MO was hired by the Ministry of Information initially to monitor public opinion in upcoming parliamentary by-elections. It soon also began to investigate the public response to the Ministry's stilted propaganda poster campaign launched in the opening months of the war. MO embarked on regularly collecting reports from observers on the main topics of the war. Directives were sent out asking for views on major war policies such as the evacuation of children from the cities (due to fear of bombing), rationing, war savings, and the blackout and the usual range of MO interests in sport, music, religion, shopping, and leisure.[16]

Many of the early observations by Mass Observers made it into the book *War Begins*. This book was published while Neville Chamberlain was still wartime prime minister and before the Blitzkrieg invasion of France, Belgium, and Holland. *War Begins* shows that the first few months of war led to public bewilderment over the "Phoney War" and the lack of the expected air raids. Despite the absence of an aerial apocalypse, *War Begins* points to a country beset by blackout and upset by wartime evacuation.[17] The evacuation of urban children to the countryside was shown as a massive failure leading to major class divisions (the authors note some middle-class rural hosts saw their working-class evacuees as "an animal threat" representing social revolution). So bad was the class hostility that three-quarters of the children went back to the cities by spring 1940.[18] The book anticipates the wartime change in government by clearly pointing out the overall lack of support Chamberlain had as a wartime leader.[19]

---

16. Heimann, *Most Offending Soul Alive*, 156–58; James Hinton, *The Mass Observers: A History, 1937–1949* (Oxford University Press, 2013), 27; 153–57.

17. Mass-Observation, *War Begins at Home*, ed. Thomas Harrisson and Charles Madge (London: Chatto and Windus, 1940), 221.

18. Mass-Observation, *War Begins at Home*, 336–37.

19. Mass-Observation, *War Begins at Home*, 424–25.

After Churchill became prime minister in May 1940, and when the Blitz began several months later, Tom Harrisson and MO came into their own. One of Tom Harrisson's leading colleagues, Bob (HD) Willcock, described the Blitz period as "a field day for MO."[20] Harrisson actively sought out blitzed cities (sometimes while the bombs were still falling) to monitor public responses. His report on the blitzed Midlands city of Coventry (bombed November 14–15, 1940) raised numerous hackles in government. Harrisson and his team arrived in Coventry immediately after the raid and found "more open signs of hysteria, terror, and neurosis . . . than during the whole of the past two months together in all areas."[21] Thirty years after the end of the war, Tom Harrisson returned to this material (then newly assigned to the MO Archive at the University of Sussex) when he wrote the book *Living through the Blitz* (1976). His book strongly argued against the myth of British unity during the Blitz and pointed to the fragility of public opinion.[22]

Unfortunately for MO, once the Blitz came to an end, the work began to dry up for Tom Harrisson and his organization. Harrisson was exasperating his government contacts through his unwillingness to tow the line and his general lack of respect for the authorities. By June 1941, the Ministry of Information was unwilling to grant him further contracts. Harrisson then made his way over to Naval Intelligence and used his skills to report on port security and the public opinion of dockworkers (both key issues during the war), which kept him employed until spring 1942. After that he lost his protection from conscription and was duly inducted into the army in 1942. While in the army he did help oversee the publication of *The Pub and the People* (1943), which had been based on the prewar Bolton investigations.[23] In 1944, Harrisson joined the Special Operations Executive (famous for off-the-grid special operations) and would be deployed behind Japanese lines into Borneo until the end of the war. MO continued along under the leadership of HD Willcock. It was commissioned to write a number of reports on rationing, propaganda, war production, and housing. One of their final and most interesting wartime publications was on postwar

---

20. Heimann, *Most Offending Soul Alive*, 166.

21. "Coventry," Field Report, Mass-Observation Archive as quoted by Hinton, *The Mass Observers*, 197.

22. Tom Harrisson, *Living through the Blitz* (London: Collins, 1976), 332.

23. Mass Observation, *The Pub and the People: A Worktown Study by Mass Observation* (London: Cresset Library, 1987 [rpt.]). Originally published in 1943.

plans in conjunction with the Advertising Service Guild titled *The Journey Home* (1944). By the time the war ended in 1945, MO was at a crossroads. Charles Madge had departed from the organization in 1940 as he felt that its reports on home-front morale were a form of "homefront espionage."[24] Harrisson was overseas serving in Borneo and would only briefly return to the UK before setting out for a position in Sarawak.

Mass Observation in the Postwar Period

Tom Harrisson remained in Sarawak until September 1946. After returning to England, he jumped back into his work at MO. Postwar projects were geared at earning money and included an investigation into gambling (paid for by grant from an organization against gambling), drinking habits (paid for by Guinness), and sexual morality (paid for by the *Sunday Pictorial* magazine).[25] Harrisson turned over the day-today operation of MO to HD Willcock and returned to Borneo in 1947. MO Began to concentrate on market research to keep going financially. They did marketing survey jobs for products from baby food to television sets and lots in between. Fortunately, newspapers gave MO more serious questions and the funding with which to do investigate them, such as the 1948 survey on capital punishment. From August to November of 1948, MO ran opinion polls on "attitudes to churchgoing, education, sport, leisure and the cost of living."[26]

The Coronation of Elizabeth II in 1953 provided MO with another opportunity to take the pulse of the nation. Directives were sent out and Mass Observers were also asked to write about customs for the coronation, as well as any diary entries noting the day's events. The coronation material reappeared in a 1961 book titled *Britain Revisited*, in which researchers also revisited old haunts in which they had lived and worked in Bolton. The team looked afresh at old topics such as work, voting, living conditions, pubs, vacations (especially in Blackpool) and new topics such as the rise of television.[27] In some ways, *Britain Revisited* is the last chapter of the old

24. Dorothy Sheridan, "Charles Madge and the Mass-Observation Archive," *New Formations* 44 (2001): 23.

25. Hinton, *The Mass Observers*, 335, 339, 356.

26. Hinton, *The Mass Observers*, 354.

27. Tom Harrisson, *Britain Revisited* (London: Victor Gollancz, 1961).

Mass Observation approach and leadership. Old-style MO studies were not garnering the national readership they had in their interwar heyday.

The decade of the 1960s saw MO somewhat disappear from the public eye but salvation was just around the corner. In 1969, two students looking to research wartime Britain, Paul Addison and Angus Calder, found the MO Archives lying around in heaps of dust in the basement of MO's London headquarters. Appalled by the condition of the papers and the lack of any organization, they were able to convince the University of Sussex to take the archive. Tom Harrisson, always open for a good business opportunity, gave the archive to the University of Sussex in return for being given a place to live and some financial assistance to organize the archive. By 1974, Tom Harrisson had become a professor at the University of Sussex.[28] His stint at Sussex did not last long: in 1976, while on a vacation in Thailand, Tom Harrisson and third wife were killed in a road accident.

By the 1970s, it was another Royal celebration that led to a publication not by MO but using the material they had collected from Elizabeth II's coronation. Philip Ziegler used a mixture of new observations and some of the older coronation material to write his book for the Queen's Silver Jubilee in 1977, *Crown and People*.[29] The wedding of Prince Charles and Lady Diana Spencer in 1981 was perfect for another MO foray into public opinion. There was a new directive and day-surveys for this event. The tragedy of Lady Diana's death in 1997 would similarly lead to another flurry of MO directives which would be heavily utilized in a book by James Thomas titled Diana's *Mourning: A People's History*.[30]

In the 1990s and early 2000s, MO captured the public mood once again. The fiftieth and sixtieth anniversaries of the end of World War II brought with it numerous national commemorations and many people wanting to know more about their grandparents' youth and life on the home front in general. Using its collection of wartime diaries, MO published books such as *Wartime Women: An Anthology of Women's Wartime Writing for Mass-Observation 1937–45*; *We Are at War: The Remarkable Diaries of Five Ordinary People in Extraordinary Times*; *Our Longest Days: A People's History of the Second World War*; and *Nella Last's War: The Second World War*

---

28. Hinton, *The Mass Observers*, 363.

29. Philip Ziegler, *Crown and People* (London: Collins, 1978).

30. James Thomas, *Diana's Mourning: A People's History* (Cardiff: University of Wales Press, 2002).

Diaries of Housewife, 49. This last book became a British television film in 2006, *Housewife, 49.* The film was created by, written by, and starred Victoria Wood and garnered two BAFTA awards, including one for Best Actress for Wood's portrayal of Nella Last.[31]

The work of MO has not stopped. The archive is still at University of Sussex under the direction of Dorothy Sheridan and is now called the Mass Observation Project. It has moved with the times: it has its own website with podcasts, news, and exhibitions. They have a Twitter feed. Their physical mailing address remains active, sending out directives and receiving physical mail. People continue to apply to be a Mass Observer. It is also going through a digitization project that will be made available for libraries to purchase. Throughout all of these nods to our changing technological world, MO has remained true to its original mission: to make an "anthropology of ourselves."

Mass Observation and the SUNY Oneonta Pandemic Diaries

Reconstructing the history of Mass Observation is an interesting historical exercise. However, for the purposes of this book, MO is considered as more than a curious mixing of genres in a different country during a distant time. As well as serving as the inspiration for SUNY Oneonta's pandemic diaries—both as the original web collection published online as *The Semester of Living Dangerously* and as the book, *Chronicling a Crisis: SUNY Oneonta's Pandemic Diaries*—the phenomenon of MO points to some key similarities to and differences from SUNY Oneonta's bloggers.

There are three important similarities between MO and the SUNY Oneonta pandemic diaries: First, there is the fact that pandemic diarists were chronicling a major crisis, as were the Mass Observers (especially through the war diaries). Second, both groups created a self-contained inclusive community. Third, media shaped the views of both sets of writers and added to myth making. Each point will be discussed in further detail below.

31. Dorothy Sheridan (ed.), *Wartime Women: An Anthology of Women's Wartime Writing for Mass-Observation 1937–45* (London: Mandarin, 1990); Simon Garfield, *We Are at War: The Remarkable Diaries of Five Ordinary People in Extraordinary Times* (London: Ebury Press, 2009); Sandra Koa Wing (ed.), *Our Longest Days: A People's History of the Second World War* (London: Profile Books, 2008); Richard Broad and Suzie Fleming (eds.), *Nella Last's War: The Second World War Diaries of* Housewife, 49 (London: Profile Books, 2006); Gavin Millar, Dir., *Housewife, 49*, ITV 2006.

The Second World War and the current COVID pandemic are not identical crises, but both were world-changing events. The Second World War led to the death of millions and reshaped both the politics and boundaries of Europe. While it is too early to ascertain the long-term effect of COVID, the experience of over 1 million deaths (and counting) in the US (more than both world wars combined), over 6 million worldwide deaths (and counting), yearlong lockdowns and immense economic disruption is truly epochal. When you are in the middle of enormous global historical events it is often impossible to predict how they will turn out. Many Mass Observers during World War Two, especially after Hitler's successful invasion of France, Belgium, and Holland, thought that Britain might be defeated. Pam Ashford, an unmarried woman working as a secretary in Glasgow wrote on May 29, 1940, "Certainly we are getting used to the idea of an invasion, but it is not here yet," and noted how most of her fellow employees preferred to surrender immediately if the Germans invaded.[32] Such fears would not be out of place compared to the uncertainties recorded in SUNY Oneonta's pandemic diaries. Also, just like the war diarists,' people had to get on with their lives while living through epic events. Reading the diary of Nella Last (who wrote millions of words as a diarist for MO between 1939 and 1966) fascinates as she reflects on major war events like the Blitz (including the bombing of her hometown of Barrow-in-Furness), as well as the more mundane realities of working for the Women's Voluntary Service (which helped organize welfare services during the war) and organizing her household of two adult sons and one cranky husband.[33] The ability to show how historical events unfold in real time when the outcome is not known, and people must live their lives with the events in the background is equally shared in both MO and the diaries.

Both MO and the SUNY Oneonta Pandemic Diaries helped create a sense of inclusion and community. Dorothy Sheridan has shown that MO validated its observers as writers and gave them a space to write. In this way it also created an actual community. Rather than live as atomized individuals set adrift during a major crisis, it gave them an anchor. Scholars have noted that many Mass Observers developed a bond and a sense of affinity with the editors of MO and other Mass Observers.[34] Several pandemic diary writers felt the same way. Maria Montoya, a professor at SUNY Oneonta

---

32. Pam Ashford, May 29, 1940, as quoted in Simon Garfield, *We Are at War*, 239.

33. Broad and Fleming, *Nella Last's War*.

34. Dorothy Sheridan, Street, and Bloome, *Writing Ourselves*, 230.

wrote in an April 2021 blog entry, "We are a community that cares, helps each other, collaborates, recovers, and starts again."[35] She added in a separate communication that during the pandemic, "All our relationships were screen mediated, and still something was lacking: the act of communal reflection on a global experience . . . [the SUNY Oneonta Pandemic Diaries] reminded us that we were still a community waiting to be freed from captivity, that we were all missing each other. . . . The Pandemic Diary allowed us to feel part of a community."[36]

A final more critical similarity that should be noted is that living through great events can lead to a sense of personal mythmaking and distortions. Such distortions are often exacerbated when people consider their own experience through the prism of media. Tom Harrisson explicitly pointed to this point in a 1973 interview with the *London Times*—"the only valid information for this sort of social history of war is that recorded at the time on the spot." Harrisson pointed to the dangers of "reality obliteration" under the pressures of distortion by media depictions, propaganda, and public pressure.[37] Even though the blog did record people's experiences a short time after they occurred, the speed of media dissemination in the twenty-first century may mean that every impression has been shaped in some ways. Undoubtedly, as time passes and the COVID events of 2020–21 fade into myth, this problem will be amplified. In *Living through the Blitz*, Harrisson noted "re-adjustments of memory are normal, healthy (and after suffering) essential."[38] Perhaps to move on with life such readjustments will also occur for survivors of the COVID pandemic.

Obviously, the choice of MO as the source of inspiration was sound due to the similarities just described. However, it should be noted that there are also some key differences. First, the proliferation of different forms of media has complicated the issue of forging selfhood through blogging. Second, the notion of gender has evolved considerably since the 1940s, and the diarists do not break down along easily identifiable gendered lines. Third, due to the existence of the internet and proliferation of images through

---

35. Maria Montoya, "Three Things I Learned about SUNY Oneonta: Talk to the Class of 2021," April 18, 2021, *Chronicling a Crisis: SUNY Oneonta's Pandemic Diaries*.

36. Maria Montoya, "Sense of Community during the Pandemic," July 14, 2021, email Communication with Matthew C. Hendley.

37. Tom Harrisson interview with George Hutchinson, *The Times [London]*, November 6, 1973, as quoted in Harrisson, *Living through the Blitz*, 324, 330.

38. Harrisson, *Living through the Blitz*, 322.

it, it is very possible that the individual memories transcribed within the blogs could become public memories. Each difference will also be discussed in detail below.

At first glance it seems that old-fashioned paper diaries favored by MO are the complete opposite of the new technology behind the pandemic diary blogs. Such generalizations should not be taken too far. As noted media scholar José van Dijck has pointed out, there are numerous myths about diaries that make them far closer to new technologies than we assume. Throughout history, even paper diaries were never fully private objects, nor were they always "written for one person but also by one person." Blogs with their fully public nature and often multiauthored format are not quite so different from diaries as they first appear.[39] Where they truly differ is that blogs are a hybrid technology and format. Blogs can either echo "traditional paper diaries . . . [or] morph into completely new interactive formats, firmly rooted in Internet culture." They can also "synchronize one's subjective experience with those of others." They can be archived and edited; preserved and revised all at the same time.[40] Thus, blogs like the *The Semester of Living Dangerously* take the idea of personally recording events to the next level. *The Semester of Living Dangerously* and *Chronicling a Crisis* parallel well with the current social media landscape, which creates a more complex sense of self but breaks somewhat from it. Andreas Kitzman has written that "the digital self . . . is a distributed one," which combines "the deliberate and conscious acts of an individual" with "data feeds, algorithms and inputs from other individuals and organization."[41] A key difference is that in both the blog and the book, though the bloggers did react to other media and impressions, the entries were not revised after being posted.

Gender is another major area of difference between the Mass Observers and the pandemic diarists. During the period covered by MO, most writers clearly understood gender as a binary. During the Second World War, women became more and more prominent as Mass Observers, a phenomenon not foreseen by the organization's founders. This blind spot was in spite of the fact that most of Mass Observation's full-time staff were female in the 1940s.

---

39. José van Dijck, *Mediated Memories in the Digital Age* (Stanford, CA: Stanford University Press, 2007), 67–69.

40. van Dijck, *Mediated Memories in the Digital Age*, 72.

41. Andreas Kitzman, "The Machines That Write Us: Social Media and the Evolution of the Autobiographical Impulse," in Adam Smyth (ed.), *A History of English Autobiography* (Cambridge, UK: Cambridge University Press, 2016), 422.

By the middle point of World War Two, not only did women outnumber men in the National Panel but their contributions "were longer, more regular and more detailed than those from men." Women were traditionally the ones who had written diaries, letters, and personal reports for families, so it is not surprising that they would be well suited to being regular contributors to MO. Furthermore, while women were confined to the private sphere, MO insisted that everyday life mattered. Women were encouraged to record seemingly mundane daily activities such as housework and child care, which may have led to a sense of self-validation.[42] As society evolved, social expectations and opportunities for women similarly changed. In his study of Mass Observers from the 1980s, James Hinton has noted that women used their diary entries to map out a much more complex process for achieving their own selfhood. Whereas men's entries expressed a "confident, composed, achieved selfhood," women's entries focused on "disjunctions, the obstacles, the paths not taken."[43] In these ways, the diarists at the heart of MO record distinctly gendered ideas of selfhood.

Gender is understood differently by today's generation. Binaries have given way to nonbinaries. It cannot be assumed that there was a simple division of male and female among the pandemic diary writers. What is extremely interesting is that perhaps due to more nuanced notions of gender, the responses generated in the diaries are equally nuanced. Unlike the stark gender divide of selfhood shown in the 1980s MO diaries by James Hinton (which can be echoed in MO diaries from other periods), the response to the COVID crisis by the pandemic diarists seems more universal. There is very little masculinized confident composed selfhood within the pandemic diary entries. Contributors of all genders to the diary focus on disjunction and disruption, isolation, impact on family, relationships, and ever-present illness and death.

One last difference that should be noted is due to the acceleration of technology and the proliferation of the internet and the importance of images found within the blogs. Most of the images shared with the pandemic diary blog were captured by cell phone cameras. There are literally billions of phones now present on the earth. The omnipresence of cell phones and the ease with which images can be captured and shared has had a massive historical impact. The ability of a cell phone to capture the

---

42. Calder and Sheridan, *Speak for Yourself*, 151.

43. James Hinton, *Seven Lives from Mass Observation: Britain in the Late Twentieth Century* (Oxford, UK: Oxford University Press, 2016), 216.

murder of George Floyd and widely share the horrific images launched a national reckoning with racial injustice in the United States. The authors of the book *Save As . . . Digital Measures* have argued that "the mobile phone is accelerating our ability rapidly to transform our personal impressions into public memories independent of the individual." They argue that this change has created a type of memory they call "memobilia [which is a] . . . form . . . enmeshed with a record of the self that traverses the usual binaries between the private and the public."[44] It is pretentious to assume that any of the images found in *Chronicling a Crisis* will become so iconic that they will somehow become widespread public memories of this period. However, it is certainly possible that on a smaller scale the SUNY Oneonta community's reading of the blogs will ensure that some of the images privately taken but shared through the medium of the blog and this book will become part of the public COVID memory of this community. The ability to do this marks a huge difference with Mass Observation's structure in which individuals submitted written diaries with no real ability to easily submit personally recorded images (although sometimes they did collect leaflets and ephemera). In addition, none of these entries would be readily or immediately shared with other community members, so that the ability of any given individual to help shape the public memory of members of their own community was nonexistent.

SUNY Oneonta was one small community living through a global crisis. However, the creators of *The Semester of Living Dangerously* and *Chronicling a Crisis* felt it was vital to use the medium of blogging to bear witness and record its impact on faculty, staff, and students. MO served as our guiding inspiration. It was born in crisis and being in a predigital age, took a different format and had some striking differences. Nevertheless, as this conclusion argues, there were enough similarities that make an extended discussion of the experience of Mass Observation very worthwhile.

---

44. Anna Reading, "Memobilia: The Mobile Phone and the Emergence of Wearable Memories," in Joanne Garde-Hansen, Andrew Hoskins, and Anna Reading (eds.), *Save As . . . Digital Measures* (Houndmills, UK: Palgrave Macmillan, 2009), 90–91.

From Pixels to Paper

Building Blog and Book

ED BECK AND DARREN D. CHASE

Most of the editorial team for *Chronicling a Crisis* was already in place by the time library director Darren D. Chase asked instructional designer Ed Beck to join the team. At that time, the institution was in the process of pivoting from nearly all its classes taught face to face, to every class being taught online using video conferencing tools. Back in the spring of 2020, the editorial team was still thinking of the pandemic diaries project as a physical archive, a collection of pages and diaries that would be gathered in our library archive and special collections, cataloged, indexed, and made available to researchers and scholars. The editorial team asked the Teaching, Learning and Technology Center was if they had any ideas about how to create a digital edition of the archive to be kept and stored in parallel to the physical collection. Fortunately, SUNY Oneonta's Teaching, Learning and Technology Center had been preparing for these types of projects for a while and had quietly been building up the internal infrastructure that the final project would need.

SUNY Oneonta had been piloting a "Domain of One's Own" initiative that had been locally branded as SUNY Create. SUNY Create was established with grant funds in 2019 as a way to promote the creation of digital learning spaces for sharing and collaboration. At its core, the vision was for a robust, supported digital ecosystem that encouraged the creation of knowledge, sharing of ideas, and participation in larger, interdisciplinary conversations on the open web. The original web collection, published online as *The Semester of Living Dangerously* does an excellent job living up to the ideals and illustrating the potential of using open web publishing tools to create an atmosphere of sharing.

When SUNY Oneonta started the SUNY Create project, and invited faculty, staff, and students to build public-facing websites on the open web, it was an act of faith in the creativity, adaptability, and responsibility of our faculty and students. What does it mean for the SUNY Oneonta and State University of New York logos proudly displayed at the bottom of our website? What stance is the institution putting forward when library and instructional design supports that are traditionally used in classes are made available for a faculty project that is not part of any one class? It is a statement of the type of institution that we want to be that institutional resources and branding should be used to enable academic projects for and by the Oneonta Community. The project grew over time from the idea of an engaged faculty member who convinced the rest of their department, who brought the dean on board, who enlisted the help of the Milne Library and the Teaching, Learning and Technology Center to build an online repository of the moment.

This book was built from those online diaries through a partnership with SUNY Press. Indeed, driving concerns of the project orbited around the modality shifts as it moved from conceptualization to implementation, and finally to preservation. Originally conceived, the project would have been a physical archive. Then it was reimagined as a digital living document, and finally it was preserved as an open access book. Moving between these modalities—from online group blog to book—required that the editorial team map and identify the gaps and bridges between the frameworks of each. Though the journal entries are the same in each modality, the framings and access points of the content are quite different. Shifting from one to the other required attention to the details of function—how will the reader experience the work? The reader experience needed to be consistent, and the affordances and value-added aspects of both modalities needed to be understood.

In the Introduction, Ann wrote about how the project transformed over time, from her initial spark of an idea to what this project eventually became. The transformation was not just a transformation of scale, as more people came on board, but also a transformation of intent. As Ed sent prototype after prototype to the collaborators, the vision began to change, from a physical archive that might have a digital component, to a digital-first project, where participants posted publicly their day, their thoughts, musings, or fears. The public nature of what we created no doubt changed what was written about and how it was shared. The imagery of pandemic, often uploaded to the blog in black and white comes to mind as the type of post that the digital format enabled.

All members of the editorial board brought their own expertise and influenced the development of the project through the lens of our professions. Both the Library and the Teaching, Learning and Technology Center were simultaneously inside and outside their traditional roles as we supported this project. The History faculty members' focus was on the public history of the moment. The library took that concept and added an emphasis of archiving and use of digital humanities tools. The Teaching, Learning and Technology Center provided the digital infrastructure, design, and support along with an intellectual bias toward open publishing and open access. The collaborative nature between our units, each with specific goals and intellectual traditions, provides a template for colleges and universities interested in fostering digital humanities.

What intellectual stances from our training, from our professions, and from our identity as members of the academic community translate into action? Mass Observation is the foundation of *Chronicling a Crisis*, but what other influences were layered on that ideological understructure? One clear influence was the movement of open publishing, not just in the fact that we were creating a public archive, but also that we were committed to providing the platform to our entire community, minimizing gatekeeping, and letting our community dictate the direction of the project. We didn't know at the time that Oneonta would become an epicenter of the pandemic in New York and be the only college in New York State—after only the first few weeks of the fall 2020 semester—to send everyone home and keep them home. As much as we sought to sustain an open and permissive platform, we worried and fretted as editors that something would be posted that would force our hands as censors. Our community shared so much, sometimes whimsical, sometimes raw, and we never had cause to remove an entry. Our trust in the Oneonta community was rewarded.

As we tinkered with the workflow and display of the website, we focused on ways to streamline the experience of both the authors and editorial team. Institutional support from one of the deans of the college and the chief information officer were key to getting our prototype connected to the SUNY Oneonta Single Sign-On. With that support from IT, every member of the community could log in with their existing credentials, have an account automatically created for them, and immediately begin writing and submitting an entry. Part of the project's success was making it as easy as possible to participate. Find the large red button that says "Contribute" and start typing. Using add-ons and plug-ins to WordPress, we adjusted and created new user roles, mapping them to the Single Sign-On to create the simplest user experience, reduce as many barriers to submission as we could, while creating a managed editorial workflow for the team to publish and share.

The library's role rose to prominence again as we sought to frame, analyze, and contextualize our community entries. At its core, librarianship includes the practice of building, describing, and maintaining collections that are discoverable, accessible, and sustainable. Another core practice of librarianship is connecting knowledge-seekers and information users to enriching content and resources. These practices are distributed, as libraries build and maintain networks with other libraries, and maintain interoperable systems.

The project needed a solution that would embody, cohere, connect, and associate the three anticipated material types: blogged diary entries, offline digital entries created in Word, and physical diaries that would be collected and eventually digitized. Of these three materials, it was recognized that the blog entries would likely be the greater part of the collection, and that the immediacy of the blog would mean that it would represent the entire project. To match both the spirit and intention of a mass observation project, we were committed to creating and sustaining an open and accessible collection because an open access solution would have the greatest audience reach and impact. We intended to deliver a sustainable collection because we wanted to ensure the long-term viability of the interwoven stories and ensure that it continued to be an enriching resource for researchers and scholars for many years. We recognized too that it would be best if the platform for the collection was interoperable with other systems, because the anticipated diversity of materials would be both digital and physical, and these would "live in different houses" and be represented by potentially different platforms and have different access points. Simply put, we designed for the content, the creators, the moment, and for the ages.

Many digital humanities projects are rooted in all manner of physical collections. Digital humanities practices and tools are used to unlock and mine a vast corpus, for example, or in other ways to digitize, process, and analyze. Used in many digital humanities projects, Voyant Tools is a free, online suite of text processing and analysis applications. It is useful in text mining. To be clear, we did not know we would text mine *The Semester of Living Dangerously*. We arrived at that point unexpectedly, at the stage when we were planning this book.

As noted, many digital humanities projects begin with a defined physical text or corpus that is digitized, processed, and analyzed. When we began planning this book, *Chronicling a Crisis* was entirely digital—an interweave of stories, images, entries on a WordPress blog, titled *The Semester of Living Dangerously*. It was live, too, and content was still being contributed. That is where we began: with a dynamic, digital (relative to other digital humanities projects), small and growing corpus that we wanted to encode into a book. It's kind of like doing digital humanities in reverse.

Why not? It was an exciting proposition, and one in which the editorial team saw opportunities to add value to the diary entries with background, context, and analysis (including themes analysis). Enter Voyant Tools.

The "Themes" section represents a kind of layer-cake composition that blends corpus analysis (using Voyant Tools) with reflective, contemplative entries intended to evoke mood and meaning while offering the reader an opportunity to see a cross section of the "cake" and engage its layers. Identifying themes was an iterative, multistage process. The editorial team read and reread the entries taking notes and meeting frequently to discuss matters. We shared our reflections on themes and talked about our favorite entries, and their unique qualities and the qualities they shared. Those conversations led to a spreadsheet of themes, with each editor assigning keywords and concepts to each entry. Next, each editor's keywords and theme concepts were compared and grouped together into keyword and theme concept clusters.

From the keyword and theme concept clusters were distilled a controlled vocabulary of master themes. Then Voyant Tools was used to identify the most frequently used unique words from the corpus, and those words were mapped to the master themes. When composing our themes analysis, we used Voyant Tools again to aid in the discovery of excerpts to exemplify each theme. This work in turn fueled the reflective, emotionally anchored composition of the theme entries.

Part of the rationale for taking our online project and sharing it as an open access book was thinking about the long-term sustainability of the project. A blog website requires many dynamic parts. The code must be updated, the database is a point of vulnerability, applications and extensions may stop being supported or be replaced with more modern solutions. A physical and digital book will not be the only way this project is preserved, but it is an excellent starting point.

In addition to exporting from the blog into these pages, we simultaneously began looking for options and ways to preserve the website. One of the complications of doing digital-first work is the notion that the web is constantly evolving. Our website depends on a specific version of PHP, a database, the WordPress application, and all of the other plug-ins, utilities, and themes we used to make our project run the way we wanted it to. Each one of those is a potential point of failure when we think of this project five years out, ten years out, and further into the future. To preserve the website, we need to "flatten it," pulling from the database and code an HTML website that requires no processing power to run, no database, and preserves the site exactly as it appeared in 2021. This archive of the site would be placed in our library open access repository in addition to this book. Long-term preservation of the project had to be considered if this were to be an effective archive, and the team worked hard to think about the long-term preservation of the digital project.

Learning along the Way

So, what was the secret sauce of *Chronicling a Crisis*? What follows is a set of distillations from its success that can be used as a practical fuel for other digital humanities projects: institutional readiness; an institutional culture that fosters creativity; process-oriented structure; faculty involvement and engagement; and awareness and bridging of modality differences between the online pandemic diaries and the book.

Before the project was a sparkle in Ann's eye, our institution had been preparing itself for similar projects. Not just the technological infrastructure to host a WordPress or an Omeka site—platforms like these offer easy on-ramps toward building digital collections. Just as critical were the conversations and strategizing about policy, time allocation in implementation and maintenance, and what the standard of care should be for these projects.

Have a culture that fosters and supports curiosity and experimentation. When engaged faculty come to you with a project they are excited about, run with it. It's true that not every project works out but always treat those potential collaborations seriously. Remain open to the experience without being too distracted about whether a project may or may not succeed. Not participating means either nothing will happen, or it will happen without you.

Imagining the completed workflow of the project and simplifying it aided our success. Submissions by students were entered directly in the platform, and they had full control to format, edit, and change the look and feel. That was no small matter during peak usage of the website, when many posts were coming in at once. If the editors had been responsible for reformatting, copying, or retyping posts, there would not have been the immediacy and the community that our project was able to embody. Working with publishing tools that already had hierarchical roles and publishing routines made building workflows for our team possible.

The faculty's role in making this a successful project can't be overstated. By and large, faculty brought the students. *Chronicling a Crisis* grew and succeeded because of those instructors who introduced or incorporated it into their courses. Most students participated by choice when learning about it from their instructors; others participated by assignment. No matter the talent, time, and energy that came from nonteaching team members, this project was animated by student participation and student/faculty connections. The poems, photo essays, bilingual entries, portraits, and works of art display the rich diversity of disciplines on our campus and are authentic expressions of student engagement and curiosity.

In spring 2021, the SUNY Oneonta pandemic diaries evolved from a digital collection into an edited volume to be published by SUNY Press. With this transformation came additional challenges specific to the medium and material type that we had not anticipated. While we had a basic "terms of use" statement on our website, SUNY Press needed a higher standard of approval to reprint the work in a book. A massive, complex communication campaign to the original contributors was required to get signed forms for each entry. One of our great regrets in this project was not building the permissions into the workflow from the very beginning, because of the number of contributors and great entries that we could not include in this final volume. In the end, these were the details—problems to solve.

Put another way: Ann's great idea led to a dynamic, interdepartmental partnership in designing, creating, and growing an open, shared content creation community born out of a moment in history. Put more generally, we created a platform for students, faculty, and staff together to reflect, compose, and interweave their stories of the pandemic—one with meaningful, enriching points of contact with the college's mission.

The three big takeaways for those eyeing a similar project:

1. Be willing to apply your talents and resources in unexpected ways.

2. Be deliberate in allowing the stories, the content, to shine with their own authentic vibrancy.

3. Take care to use practices, technologies, and tools in order to create a strong yet lightweight bridge between the creators, their input, and the output with connections to readers, researchers, and scholars—today, and for years to come.

Themes

DARREN D. CHASE AND MATTHEW C. HENDLEY

In this section, we will outline some recurring themes that appeared throughout the entries of the SUNY Oneonta pandemic diaries. We feel it is a necessary compositional and emotional exercise to document and reflect on patterns, layers of context and points of contact which emerge from reading and analyzing the entries. This section registers each main theme as it is felt and understood by the editors, with context from the corpus (which consists of quotations from the entries).

This section can be read in conjunction with reading the entire entries themselves or on its own.

Belief

Belief is an old word. The *Oxford English Dictionary* defines belief as "mental conviction." Belief and things believed and not believed are directly present in dozens of entries, and otherwise infuse the corpus. In the early months of the pandemic the uncertainties around COVID-19 transmission placed people outside a framework of routine and certainty.

The experiences of some put belief into sharp focus—expressing it as a fear of COVID-19 infection as seen in Hales Pink's May 2, 2020, entry, or a polar opposite belief that COVID-19 was an overstated threat, as noted by Nadia Boyea in her May 3, 2020, entry. The tension between these opposites was acutely experienced by many, and inhabiting that tension fostered other experiences of belief, some in a positive light as noted by Johnathon Shannon when he wrote, "It is my firm belief that we as human beings are a resilient species because of our ability to recover from the hardest of times, to get up, brush off the dust and dirt, and try again." Other expressions of belief were more reflective of ambiguity and uncertainty, for example, when Janice Hambor writes, "I don't know what to believe. I am afraid I am taking this too seriously. I am terrified that I am not."

Emotions

Emotions expressed by the *SUNY Oneonta Pandemic Diaries* authors were deeply felt. Sadness, joy, anger, along with a full palette of emotions colored the entries. Emotions resonate singularly or blended together, as described by Julian Gotiangco in April 2020: "Dear Diary, In case you didn't already know, I'm home from school because of the Coronavirus. All our classes will be online now. I have a lot of mixed emotions. A lot of things that I had planned got canceled."

Emotions also moved. Casey Collette experienced the looping, speeding, climbing, and falling emotions in the April 14, 2020, entry: "My great-grand-mother is still in the hospital being quarantined there while everyone in our house has been showing symptoms. It has been a roller coaster of emotions. How could something I thought was so far away affect my life this much?"

Moving in the pulsing rhythm of a turning wheel, Cordelle Abernathy describes emotions passing through pain and strife, arcing toward peace: "Worry and fear, two constant emotions for man, but through it all, Every-thing is gonna be groovy. War and disease occur but that's Nature's cycle, ya dig? This is another turn in the Wheel and a new age in the Kali Yugic cycle, but everything is still gonna be groovy. As long as we stay healthy, fit, smart, productive, and beautiful, it's all gonna be groovy."

Hales Pink reflected on the experience of emotions as a kind of intense weather—"how the world is now"—that cannot be avoided or contained but will be passed through into a less turbulent future: "It is okay to have all the feelings. Frustration, sadness, depression, anxiety, fear. But also have happiness, love, excitement, pride, enjoyment. Accepting that this is how the world is at the moment and everyone is doing their best or should be doing their best during these times is so important. We can't let ourselves get sucked into our negative emotions. Feel them, sit in them, but don't let them consume you. Life has already been turned upside down, but you're still alive, you've still got your future, so live your days for the ones you will have when this is over."

Emptiness

Feelings of emptiness are based on the recognition that individuals and the spaces they inhabit are vessels within vessels. Emptiness is revealed when the stuff drains away. Experiences of emptiness in unexpected places were described by diary authors, as when Ashley Cruz wrote in September 2020, "Once the virus broke out in the US, it reached such an effect that entire spaces in New York City were deserted, which was baffling to me, as I never imagined such places could ever be empty."

There is a poignancy to entries describing emptiness, suggesting that once layers have been stripped away only the elements and emotion remain, as seen in Michelle Hendley's October 29, 2020, entry, "The long walk I took that day was simultaneously invigorating because of the sunshine and warmth and devastating because of the emptiness and silence."

Food

Food anchored us, tethering us to life in ways that felt more meaningful and precious during the pandemic and through the dramatic changes it brought to our lives. Authors wrote of savoring meals, of meals shared, of dreaming of and missing favorite foods and restaurants. "We were going to get Chinese food for dinner, but no one answered so we made pasta and meatballs for dinner! It was so good," wrote Cassandra Snow on March 29, 2020.

Food became subject to health and safety protocols, as noted by Clifford O. Sweezey in his December 20, 2020, entry: "After coming home, my aunt would wash all the food before putting it away, something that I'm sure none of us do as of December 2020 with case counts completely blowing out those of late-March and early-April."

In her entry titled "Food for Thought," Ann Traitor reflected on the experience of food shopping in a grocery store early in the pandemic. The tension and unreality of experiencing a familiar place in an uncomfortable new context is acutely observed: "It was surreal. There were a good number of people in the store but that was not the most surprising part: it was the silence. There was no background 'music-to-shop-by,' no announcements on 'sale items fresh from the bakery,' no 'people-out-and-about' noise of any kind. The only thing we heard was the muffled shuffle of feet. Even the creaky carts were silent. No one chatted or even said 'excuse me.' Wide-eyed and fearful, people pushed their carts, looked at everyone else as a potential food-stealing enemy, and grabbed things quickly off shelves. One woman was actively crying, tears streaming down her face, as she pushed her mostly empty cart from one aisle to another. She made not a sound."

Maggie McCann registered gratitude for the food she had and considered ways that the pandemic intensifies food insecurity and the challenges of homelessness: "As terrible as this plague has been I've realized that I am very lucky. I have my family that loves me, I have food, I have a place to rest my head. There are people other there of all ages that needed the free lunch system at schools to eat daily. There are people that depend heavily on food pantries. There are people in abusive households that have been stuck there for weeks now. There are people who don't have access to their medicine. There are people who can't even hide from the monster because they don't have a home."

Freedom

Freedom is a metaphor. It is a hall of mirrors and also an object seen within the mirrors and also a spirit animating the object seen within the mirrors. As a theme, freedom is described mostly through absence and the sense that freedom is lost. "I miss driving and having my music loud with the windows down and my left hand feeling the wind, the freedom. It's literally nothing, but it's one of my simplest pleasures in life," writes Cecille Ruiz on April 20, 2020. That April marked the beginning of a kind of Season of Freedoms Lost, with nearly all of the entries that reflect on absent freedoms being written that month.

Christina Avana, like other authors, listed with bittersweet energy those freedoms she most missed: "I miss my old life, before this virus. I miss my freedom. I miss Oneonta and doing what I want when I want to. I miss seeing my friends every day and going out with them or watching movies. I miss not being told what to do or being annoyed by my siblings. I miss my independence and I cannot wait for this to be over to get that back for the remainder of the time I'm home and so on in college."

Other authors observed connections between a current loss of freedom to a previous state of loss, as described by Kathryn Kalinoski in November

2020: "I thought I didn't really have a social life before the virus, but now it really is non-existent. It doesn't help that I'm so depressed almost all of the time, and because of life, I have no actual freedom of my own."

Health

The word *health* is a child of the word *heal*, which is an old Germanic word meaning "to make whole or sound in bodily condition." The COVID-19 pandemic centered on health and health care in its myriad aspects. Concerns for bodily and mental condition received much attention in the pandemic diaries, ranging from expressions of anxiety ("COVID has exponentially increased an already existing mental health crisis amongst my generation," written by Joseph Trombetta on January 8, 2021) to warm wishes ("Tidings of staying healthy and staying at home were exchanged," written by Michelle Hendley on April 2, 2020).

"As a medical anthropologist, I think about sickness (or health) as significantly a social and cultural experience," wrote Sallie Han on May 6, 2020, in an entry titled "Let's all become armchair medical anthropologists," musing on social and public behavior as a necessary engine of culture change in overcoming the pandemic. Looking at the same horizon (returning to "normalcy") through mists of uncertainty, Tanha Rani wrote on November 5, 2020, "It feels like I don't remember much about how life was before the pandemic, but at the same time, whatever it was, I want to experience it again because I'm slowly forgetting what 'normal' really is."

History

Understandably one of the key themes that come out of the blog entries is History or History in the Making. The eight entries with this theme can be analyzed as being linked to specific events, reflections on campus history, retrospectives on history as well as reflections on the nature of history and record keeping itself. The fact that the pandemic was a global event naturally led blog writers to compare it to previous epochal events. September 11 was evoked, including in the entry "Pandemic Diaries" by Christina Avana in April 2020, where she noted it as something she did not live through but originally thought "was the worst thing that could happen." The murders of Breonna Taylor, George Floyd, and Ahmaud Arbery and resulting demonstrations for racial justice were also events referred to in the summer of the pandemic. In his blog entry, Matthew C. Hendley documents his family's presence at the Black Lives Matter protest in Cooperstown on June 7, 2020. The entry compares racial hatred and its destructiveness to that of the pandemic. The final event evoked was the election of President Biden and Vice President Kamala Harris in November 2020, in Emma Trumino's entry "A Break from the Virus." The author spoke hopefully of this event to unleash a new mood of moderation and unity in the United States. The aforementioned events are nationwide and major, but some history references were more localized. In his April 2020 entry, "20 Years in 2 weeks," Jim Greenberg noted how history was made through the rapid evolution to online instruction (after 20 years of false starts). A few entries approached history from a retrospective angle. Bill Simons in his August 2020 entry considered baseball history and online trivia contests as a route to "staying centered" and continuing a sense of camaraderie. Ann Traitor in her November 2020 entry "Three Little Words" considered the phrase "my fellow Americans" as a clarion call throughout American history for unity and common purpose and feared the pandemic was undermining it. Other history-minded entries reflected on the nature of history and record keeping itself. Many blog editors felt a compelling need to document these times. This feeling was echoed by the editors of this book: the deep human feeling of the need to collect material and document the unique time the bloggers were living through. The pandemic diary entry "We Used to Wait" by Matthew C. Hendley reconsiders the old-fashioned paper letter. It wonders if the pandemic might lead to a revival of this medium of communication much revered by historians and posits that letter writing can be "both therapeutic and meaningful" in a moment of crisis to keep the historical record going and reach out to individuals.

Home

Home is "the place where a person or animal dwells." Pandemic diary authors wrote of being stuck at home or quarantining away from home and family. Living, working, and staying at home brought some challenges and some joy, such as surprising opportunities to become closer to friends and family. Dullness and isolation were other experiences of living and working at home, as expressed with clarity by Cecille Ruiz in her April 20, 2020, entry: "I am so bored at home and so tired of seeing the same four faces every day."

In a similar vein, Christina Avana described the struggles of home and family and the loss of the safety and comforts of living on campus in her April 2020 entry: "I miss school and I miss my friends. Being stuck at home for this long is torture. Having contact with my family only causes nothing but fights, it's horrible. I miss my old life. College was my safe place."

Justice/Injustice

Justice and the element found in its absence, injustice, are the stuff of law, equity, and rights. In their posts, the *SUNY Oneonta Pandemic Diaries* authors sought to align the pressures and demands of the pandemic with what is fair, what is equitable with what is just. The dimensions of justice, fairness and equity were experienced both publicly and privately, as were the many points of contact between them. "How does one protest during a pandemic?" asked Matthew C. Hendley in a June 7, 2020, entry that reflected on COVID-19 impacts on the terms of engagement for social and racial justice activism, public action, and protest.

The impacts and stresses of the pandemic gave a distinct shading to injustice, as Makayla Zambrano considered when she wrote on November 29, 2020, "All SUNY schools deserve to be treated the same but that is not what's happening. This virus has made me realize one thing: life is not fair at all."

"No one is passing through this time unscathed," wrote Susan Goodier on January 12, 2021, in an entry reflecting on her private reckoning with injustice as being nevertheless a shared and perhaps inescapable challenge each individual must face; COVID-19 times making us all together alone in coming to terms with the weight of injustice and the sharpness of global angst.

Life

Life is the animating force. We have it, we lose it. We measure it, we reflect on those things that give it meaning. It begins, it is, then it ends. The SUNY Oneonta pandemic diaries observed and felt tensions between living and dying, expressions of life and the concern or fear that it had been too much altered—too shifted from "normal." Victoria Chicolo in her April 6, 2020 entry asks: "**Imagine** if life doesn't get back to normal? Is this life the new normal?" Her questions are representative of many authors questioning the meaning of life during a deadly pandemic.

For Cindi Hall, as with other authors, the challenges of the pandemic intensified anxieties to a degree that they encompassed a life out of control: "I have anxiety and my heart races just with thoughts of dreaded things that are upcoming. I am older and this just started recently in the past 3 years because of many things in my life that are just not controllable. I have always been a 'fixer' and I cannot 'fix' what is going on around me today; this causes me sleepless nights and crying jags."

Life is often described as a journey. Though we may plan our trip and chart our destination, authors like Maria Cristina Montoya observed how the pandemic led to detours and unexpected turns and twists: "I feared discrimination and the social nightmare that most of us escaped when we decided to cross the border. I even suffered through the idea I had to leave again; I am too old for another exile journey. But today, after a day of symbolism, and a final happy episode, I feel immense gratitude by having earned a piece of land in the north, with water, a family, and surrounded by good people, 'hombres y mujeres de bien.'"

Loss

Loss permeates the SUNY Oneonta pandemic diaries. Authors observe and represent in their work a whole world of loss: lost time, lost freedom, lost connections to others, lost health, lost life, lost happiness. One year into the pandemic, in March 2021, Ann Traitor observed an experience of loss bound also by another loss, reflecting on the deaths of friends and family and how survivors lost also the moments to come together, grieve together, and share a farewell: "Death seemed to stalk me. I started to dread looking at my email or getting a phone call from a relative. For whom is 'Death' the last friend now, escorting my loved ones away? The first one was the hardest. The shock factor really hit home. My work kept me sane. I buried myself in books and work to keep my mind off of the loss, off of the lack of the funeral, off of the idea that the ashes were in a can in a "holding room," waiting to be picked up at some future, unspecified time. I told myself that others have it worse, be grateful for what still remains."

In her April 14, 2020, entry, Jillian Martelle showed optimism in the face of loss, sensing support and strength to overcome it: "There is no point in worrying for the future when we don't focus on the present. We will all get through this. There will be sad times and losses, but there will also be courage and strength. In a time like this, no one is alone even if it feels that way. We are all going through this together and we will all come out stronger because of it. We just have to have hope."

Masks

On April 3, 2020, the Centers for Disease Control (CDC) first recommended wearing a mask to help lessen the transmission of COVID-19. New York Governor Andrew Cuomo issued an executive order requiring masking on April 15, 2020. On July 14, 2020, the CDC issued a press release calling on all Americans to wear masks to prevent COVID-19 spread. Though it was not the case in the early days of the pandemic, by early April 2020, mask wearing was recommended in order to lessen the spread of the virus. By May 2020, most authors wore masks. At times masks were unavailable. Darren D. Chase, like other authors, found creative solutions for creating improvised masks, including borrowing his dog's bandanas: "With recent advice encouraging the wearing of face masks in public, Cosima's bandana wardrobe is being repurposed. Thank you, Cosima, for your sweetness and love, and thank you for the face masks."

Masking was divisive and politicized, and tensions and conflict around masking were observed. Author Melissa Marietta wrote expansively on those tensions in her entry titled "The time my kid took off her mask at Target": "The young woman, two dozen paces from us, stood firm, her feet planted in a power stance, her arms waving, and her eyes blazing above her mask. 'There's a pandemic happening! Put on a mask! What is wrong with people?' "

Milestones

Although history and historical milestones matter, most people also mark their lives with personal milestones that revolve around birthdays, graduations, and seasonal holidays. Three entries in particular make noted reference to such personal details. For the most part it is the inability to mark such rituals that makes such poignant reading.

Early in April of 2020, in "Socialization," Maggie McCann notes the inability to hold a large family party for her cousin's birthday and remembers fondly family gatherings and barbecues. Even more evocative is Melissa Lavin's short and pointed blog entry just after Halloween 2020. Titled "Pandemic Halloween Is a Ghost Town," she notes how few children came by to trick or treat but how a few brave souls yearned for normality, for candy and to have their costumes admired. As Melissa noted. "In a pandemic, Halloween is by ghosts in a ghost town." Perhaps the most succinct but meaningful post is from May 2020. Titled "The End" by Kim Se-Chan, it shows a picture of someone looking out of a dorm window waiting to leave after exams.

Nature

"Other animals are blissfully ignorant to the social distancing rule," wrote Gabrielle Bush on April 14, 2020. During the pandemic diary authors saw nature unbound and thriving in neighborhoods and spaces left vacant of human activity. As housebound days increased, authors felt an imperative to go outdoors. Once there, nature was experienced, appreciated, and observed through a new lens. For Gabrielle Bush (again) nature was an escape: "Meanwhile it seems as though people are making the time to get outside and enjoy nature, an escape from the quarantine.

Observing how quickly animals filled spaces unoccupied or unthreatened by people, Matthew C. Hendley wrote in May 2020: "We have always assumed that we had the freedom to go anywhere. We had machines and large brains. Animals had to adapt to us. We watched them and they hid from us. The pandemic has flipped the script. Now we hide and they watch us. Perhaps the wild ones were the wise ones all along."

In other reflections on nature, Matthew C. Hendley one month later saw connections between the workings of nature and the workings of society, recording a sense that racial hatred spreads like a virus: "Biological diseases are caused by nature and spread by people. Racial hatred is fanned by people and spread by people. If a nation can come together to conquer one, why can't they conquer the other as well?"

New York (NYC, Oneonta)

Geography and a sense of place pervades a number of entries in the pandemic diaries. Eight entries are strongly linked to New York as a geographic entity (whether represented as New York City, Oneonta, or other localities). As about 40 percent of SUNY Oneonta's students are from the New York City and

Downstate area, it is unsurprising that references to this area are strong. The entry by Maggie McCann titled "April 1, 2020" evokes the feeling of being in the epicenter of the pandemic in which many in her immediate circle of family and friends were testing positive. In it, she expresses thankfulness of her ability to go for a short drive and walk in nearby Lemon Creek Park in Staten Island. Photographic references to New York City abound in the blogs. "Empty NYC" by Joseph Suhovsky portrays the eeriness of walking through a now empty city with shuttered theaters and minimal foot traffic. The remaining blogs portray New York outside of the metropolis. Jaclyn Kennedy's COVID journal from September 2020 notes of her activities in Oneonta must have been fairly typical for students. The number of positives skyrocketed when classes began in fall 2020, leading to the shutdown of the campus. Jaclyn notes how seemingly innocent activities like going out to dinner in Oneonta early in the semester led to multiple friends getting sick, including herself. Shasha Wallis's "Pandemic diary" entry refers to trying to cope and socialize safely in her unnamed small town in Upstate New York and bonding with friends in her last summer before college began. As she wrote "we created our own bubble with our eight-person friend group."

Relationships

Friends, family, coworkers, relationships—these were major themes of the SUNY Oneonta pandemic diaries. Isolation fueled a fear of losing connections to relationships. Authors like Julia Perrone reflected on the dearness of our connections to one another: "A hug from a friend, a meal with your family, and the simple exchange of please and thank you are all such minuscule things. But they are so important, and the simple things are the key to happiness. Things that used to be important to me aren't any more like shopping, makeup, and how I'm gonna get my crush to like me back. Materialistic things are not important, and nothing is more powerful than strong relationships between family and friends."

The pandemic led to conditions that lead to innovations in our connections to friends, family, and others. Michelle Hendley described how her extensive and far-flung family stayed connected in her April 2, 2020, post: "In response to the coronavirus pandemic, one of my many cousins set up a WhatsApp chat group for our family so that we can stay in touch during this time. I have at least 25 first cousins on my father's side of the family, most of whom are on the chat group. Many of my cousins are parents and grandparents. The family is very large and scattered across the world: Jamaica, the country where my cousins, grandparents, parents, aunts, uncles, siblings and I were born, Canada, Australia, the United Kingdom, and the United States."

School

Semesters are measures of time at college, a term, and a period. The *SUNY Oneonta Pandemic Diaries* authors wrote on a broad range of experiences and thoughts, each a focal point in the movement of a scope directed at school. The scope focused on many things: family, self, health, emotions; as it reveals each thing, there perhaps distant and blurry—but present—was school.

Many authors described the dramatic changes brought by the pandemic and the rapid pivot to online school, and the experience of it, and how it influenced feelings about school. Julian Gotiangco wrote on April 4, 2020: "I had a weird epiphany lately. I'm getting ahead of myself here. I'm looking forward to the end of the school year, but when the summer break ends, for the first time, I'm not going to be upset that I'll be going back to school. This is really the first time I can say I miss school and I wish I could be there. Classes started yesterday. I'll put in another entry when this first week is over."

Others expressed a pervasive numbness in the face of the isolation and other challenges brought by the pandemic, as expressed by Franklyn Macario in his single-sentence entry titled "Frozen": "Everything seems to be Frozen. Our social lives, school, work, roads, parks, and the world in general. Everything is Frozen."

Seasons

Seasons moved from background to foreground of awareness throughout the SUNY Oneonta pandemic diaries.

In entries the season became the main dish, hungrily anticipated as seen in Lexi Veitch's entry titled "Craving Spring": "Every year, at the end of a long winter, I crave for the blooming of flowers and the return of birds to fill the air with songs. Spring is coming, but it feels as if it is crawling to the start line. Spring brings new beginnings and thoughts of rejoicing with friends and family at picnics or baseball games. But as I think about everything that should be happening, I am reminded about what is yet to come."

Self

Through the process of describing or considering our relationships to ourselves, the "self" becomes an other. From self-criticism to self-love, authors came to terms with themselves in the frame of the pandemic. Joseph Trombetta, like a number of authors, reflected on working against himself in his January 8, 2021, entry: "We can all be our own worst enemy. Self-criticism is an act of sabotage against oneself. To an extent, it can be useful in developing yourself as a person, and I still engage in it. However, certain things are out of your control. During fall of 2019 I criticized myself for quandaries that I had no real control over."

Identity is mutable. It finds shape within the current and period of our lives. When it changes, we might fail to recognize ourselves, or dislike who we see. We might also love the self we meet, as described by Danielle D. in her April 8, 2020, entry: "My favorite part of this experience was getting to spend time with myself. I am finding self-love and am actively caring for myself better. I also have been working on my compassion skills with my family as we haven't always had the greatest relationship."

Social Distance

Social distance is the invisible bubble around an individual in a shared space that is intended to protect a person's health by reducing the risk of the spread of the infection from person to person. Authors reflected on the dimensions of social distance were both an established, measurable six feet, and an immeasurable emotional distance; these were sometimes mapped to the same space and/or moment, as observed by Maggie McCann on March 28, 2020, "It's been a week since people have been moving their stuff out of their dorms, my friends across the hall have all moved their things out except for Kiara, it's a ghost town on campus, everyone's keeping their distance, getting in and out as fast as we can."

Molly Jean Feulner poignantly recorded social distance in her photo essay titled "Quarantined;from the outside looking in," writing, "I think they are enjoying the routine and familiarity of the content, but I can see in their eyes that they are confused and somewhat sad by the distance."

Other authors like Matthew C. Hendley, reflected on the irony of social distancing in social schemes already defined by its opposite; in his case, the collective action of protest: "There was a deep irony at work as we protested during the pandemic. Social distance and masks were used by the protesters as a conscious way to avoid the contagion of COVID."

Social Interactions

"Social Interactions" as a theme is infused within the SUNY Oneonta pandemic diaries, and explicitly addressed by some authors. Infused, it is sometimes expressed as the tension felt when social interactions are pulled away or suspended in the space of social distancing: "The experience of social distancing and self-quarantines have taken a toll on everyone I know in one way or another," wrote Nadia Boyea on April 11, 2020.

More pointedly, Jillian Martelle expressed frustration that this was a time when people should be together: "This is a time when people should be coming together, but instead, the entire world is shutting themselves inside their houses and locking their doors."

With a different, hopeful tone, Sallie Han reflected on how the pandemic has brought her children closer together: "So, my hope is that years from now, they will look back at this time and remember not just the strangeness and sadness of this moment and spending so much time on screens and missing their friends, but also that they got to be together and enjoy having a brother/sister who would walk, ride bikes, sing along to the same songs. So, maybe that will be a happy memory from now."

Raymond Scalfani described social interactions as being within a home-grown health and safety protocol when he wrote on January 8, 2021, "My housemates and I decided to make an agreement with one other house that we were only allowed to see each other so that we could still have that social interaction that was outside of our immediate household."

Stagnation

Many bloggers kept up a sense of optimism or displayed resilience. However, for others the mood was one of stagnation and emptiness. This is especially evident in seven entries, in which the emotion of feeling frozen or trapped looms large. Franklyn Macario put it best in his April 2020 blog "Frozen": "Everything seems to be Frozen. Our social lives, school, work, roads, parks, and the world in general. Everything is Frozen." The sameness of every day is another subtheme linked to stagnation. Kelly N. Tenbus in her April 2020 entry "What day is it?" felt bored and that "Nothing feels productive or rewarding. A day starts and ends, but nothing has changed." Feelings of loss and delay amid the stagnation also feature widely. For several bloggers this is tied to health concerns. Sven Anderson, a long-time professor in the Art Department wrote in his August 2020 entry, "The View from Here," about his great plans for a fall 2020 sabbatical that would have involved travel in Iceland, Scandinavia, Canada, and Alaska. As he had a disease affecting his lungs, he was forced to abandon his plans and instead stay at home and "Sit and think and sit and stare." The main breaks to his feelings of stagnation were observing nature and wildlife around him and doing artwork based on pictures from his memory. Julia Harkins in April 2020, who suffers from severe asthma, also wrote of her feelings of isolation and stagnation. Rather than making memories at school, "I sit in my house and hear from almost no one, which is a huge reality check." Reading blogs focused on stagnation shows the major mental health impacts of the pandemic.

Technology

During a pandemic in which so much work was online and social relations were often conducted on screens, contemplations about technology were a steady theme in fourteen blog posts. The main subthemes that emerged surrounding technology revolved around opinions about online teaching and learning (by both students and professors), social media and social ties, and technology as a distraction. Online instructors were relatively sanguine and sometimes enthusiastic when addressing the new medium. Susan Goodier in "As COVID-19 semester # 2 draws to a close . . ." at the end of fall 2020, celebrated the ability to bring in outside experts to her class via Zoom (including the author of one of the books read by her students). Jim Greenberg in "20 Years in 2 weeks" noted that SUNY Oneonta had suddenly embraced the same online learning it had previously viewed it with skepticism. Students were generally more pointed in their criticisms of technology and online learning. Lexi Veitch in "Learning" noted that her childhood bedroom had become the equivalent of "the library, dorm room and gym" and that her "productivity comes in waves." Strongly negative student emotions toward online learning were voiced by Makayla Zambrano who wrote in "Being Positive" in October 2020 of being unmotivated and having massive headaches at the end of online lectures. She was hoping strongly for on-campus courses in the future, since other SUNY schools had managed it even during the pandemic. One month later in "Last 8 am of the Semester," Makayla noted that although online learning had some positives (including going to class in her pajamas and sleeping in later on class days) she was not retaining as much information as she would in person and that she hoped for "an in person . . . quality education" in the fall. Not all blogging about technology is concerned with education. A good number of posts pointed to social media and the social ties that technology attempted to foster. Joseph Trombetta in his January 2021 post "My Life Before and Now" pointed out that video chats especially (but not text messaging) were relatively successful at maintaining "human social engagement." Matthew C. Hendley's post "We Used to Wait" compared the instantaneous communications made possible by modern social media and mobile phones with the calming aspects of old-fashioned letter writing. He lamented the shallowness of modern technologies and the anxiety that they created. Ed Beck's post "Doomscrolling" from November 2020 also points to anxiety fueled by social media. Technology allowed him to check the *New York Times* online COVID tracker ten times per day. Finally, technology has been used as a distraction. Gabrielle Stoetzner noted in her April 2020 entry "Quarantine quietness" that she formerly used social media as a distraction to deal with boredom, but COVID news only made her more anxious. Consequently, she changed to other more practical tasks and even took to napping. Sierra Autumn Gold in her entry "Impulse Spending" tells of her addiction to online shopping, which culminated in her purchase of a new Xbox to help pass the time. The technology blogs reveal that the new online world was neither wholly utopian nor wholly dystopian.

Time

Time is the most highly used word in the SUNY Oneonta pandemic diaries. Time can be many things or nothing. It can be known by its movement or by its stillness. Time has been defined in the *Oxford English Dictionary* as "a nonspatial continuum in which events occur in apparently irreversible succession from the past through the present to the future."

Time moved slowly for the many students and faculty enduring the COVID pandemic. Unsurprisingly time was a major theme among eight blog entries. Some of the time-related subthemes that were most prominent in the pandemic diaries included ideas around the passage of time, the future, and the interruption of time. As people waited out the virus (sometimes in actual quarantine or near-quarantine-like conditions) bloggers became very aware of the passage of time. Tyra A. Olstad in May 2020 literally wrote about "Measuring a month" and admitted "days and weeks have blurred together." To make sense of the endlessly similar days she took to making calendar notes of weather or wildlife spottings. In April 2020, Ethan Teper, a student on the autism spectrum, noted in "What Message would this give me ten years ago?Ago" that traumatic events from his past were resurfacing. He thought he had put these memories behind him, and he was working toward resolution. However, he now felt all this progress had been made useless due to the rapid shutdowns from the pandemic. The future and fears over the future were also a prominent theme. Several bloggers had very fearful views of the future. In "A Dark Winter Ahead," Emma Trumino wrote in November 2020 about fears of a second wave of the virus arriving before a vaccine became available. Earlier in the pandemic, in April 2020, Cindi Hall wondered in "These times are not for people with anxiety!"whether things would ever return to normal and whether she might die and not able to live to see her grandchildren grow up. Three entries from April 2020 also consider the idea of the future from multiple perspectives. Victoria Chicolo wrote poignantly in April 2020 about imagining the future and ponders "Is this life the new normal?" She wonders if anyone truly understands how the future will pan out. Lexi Veitch looked to the future as the change of seasons. She mentions her cravings for spring and with it "the blooming of flowers and the return of birds to fill the air with songs." Wesley Bernard, a professor in the Art Department, spoke of the despair and resilience his students had shown and posits that the nation is most likely "ascending" in the future and not "descending." The interruption of time is another intriguing theme. Maria Cristina Montoya's August 2020 post "Where did I leave off?" expresses the feeling of the usual flow of the academic year interrupted though notes. "It has been the longest summer break at home with my family." Time was ever present in many of the blogs as people waited out the pandemic.

Work and Telecommuting

Even during the pandemic work was unavoidable and appeared as a popular theme among the bloggers. Work evolved; some people lost their jobs but

work itself endured. Some of the themes in the eleven blog entries most
relevant to the theme of work include the differences of working from home
and its privileges, the changes to work wrought by technology, work guilt,
the demands of academic work, and money pressures from loss of work.
One of the biggest divides in the US during the pandemic was between
those who were able to work from home and those who were not. Sallie
Han put it best when she noted in her post "Let's all become armchair
medical anthropologists" that "Those of us who have the privilege of doing
so have made extraordinary changes by living in 'lockdown' and 'shelter in
place' and adapting our activities to enable work and school from home."
Molly Jean Feulner's post "Quarantined; from the outside looking in" contained interviews from multiple local people. One of her interview subjects
(also named Molly) from Westville, New York, noted how "fortunate" she
was to be able to work from home though her work became much more
challenging. Another subject from Milford, NY, named Karla, shared her
gratitude at being able to work from "a safe and loving home environment."
Other bloggers reflected on the different sensations of working from home.
Darren D. Chase's post "Careful &Precise" revealed his curiosity about the
work environments of his colleagues. He wondered if they could smell fresh
brewed coffee, were working alone or had others in the house. Workplace
challenges due to newfound reliance on technology were often voiced. One of
Molly Jean Feulner's interviewees named Kerstin Green spoke of a different
set of technological challenges. She worked as director of a private nursery
school and kindergarten online with twenty-five young children. It was
immensely difficult to keep her charges learning and on task while online.
Perhaps better with technology and certainly more neatly organized was
Maria Cristina Montoya. Her photo entry "My office during quarantine"
shows an immaculate and well-planned home working space. No matter what
the work environment is, some bloggers feel they could always be doing
more. Sallie Han in an April 2020 post titled "I'm Falling Down On My
Ethnographic Responsibilities and I Need To Be OK With That"laments
her inability to launch a major ethnographic project to collect data from
distinct groups such as pregnant women during COVID. She pushes back
on this work guilt and reflects on how stretched thin she already is.

The final work themes that are worth highlighting show the huge
amount of stress students and others faced. Academic work from students
and the stresses they suffer from (often while also having to do paid work
to pay their bills) looms large. In the entries "Fitness and Quarantine" and
"April Showers bring . . . a boatload of work!"Cordell Abernathy lists the

many home tasks and work tasks that must be done. Similarly, Cecille Ruiz in "Another Thursday . . ." and Clifford O. Sweezey in "My COVID Experience" confess to the manifold pressures of academic and paid labor. Cecille Ruiz especially notes "financial stress" from the work instabilities her family experienced due to COVID. Molly Jean Feulner's interviewees mention losing jobs and going through partial unemployment. To conclude, it is unsurprising that many bloggers looked forward to the end of the new world of work they were experiencing. The urge to return to a more normal working schedule is revealed by Cecille Ruiz in her other post, "Introduction . . ." in which she notes both her dedication to hard work and desire to return to normality—"I worked two jobs on campus, back when we were still on campus. I miss my jobs, sometimes. I prefer working in real life as opposed to this whole virtual reality life I feel like I'm in. I hope things go back to normal soon." The urge for a return to normality and the reassurances of a familiar work environment were a common theme for most work-centered blog posts.

Index